TABLE OF CONTENTS

INTRODUCTION

Fleas and ticks are the most common ectoparasites affecting companion animals. They can cause dermatitis, pruritus, skin infections, allergic reactions and anemia. Additionally, these pests have been associated with the transmission of zoonotic disease causing organisms such as *Rickettsia* and *Bartonella*. Their impact is not limited to companion animal health and human health but also includes significant economic consequences due to the financial resources allocated to their control.

It is much easier to achieve the goal of not seeing adult fleas on a pet than it is to prevent an occasional unseen flea from biting a pet and causing itching. This concept can be difficult to accept in a flea-scarce environment.

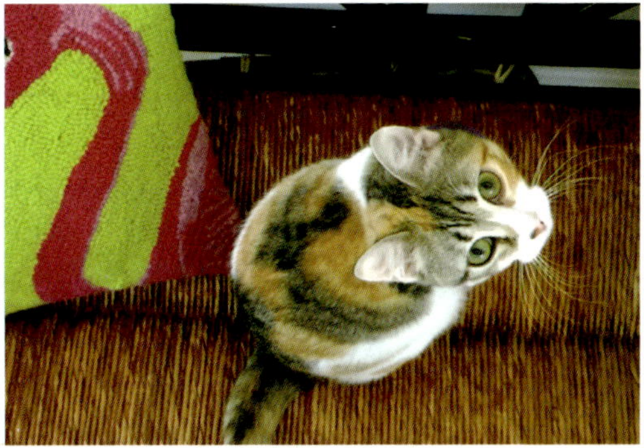

Keeping a pet free of fleas and ticks is easier and less expensive than treating a pet and the environment once an infestation has occurred. This is particularly true if a pet is flea allergic. Image courtesy of Dr. Natalie Isaza and the Veterinary Community Outreach Program at the University of Florida, US.

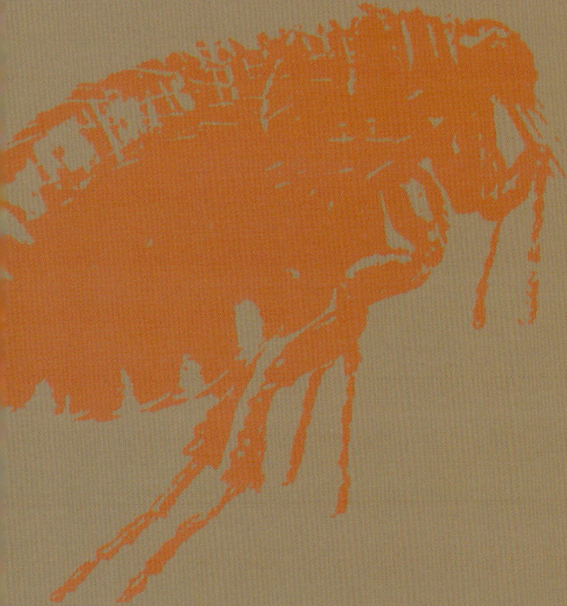

FLEAS

Dunbar Gram
DVM, DACVD, MRCVS

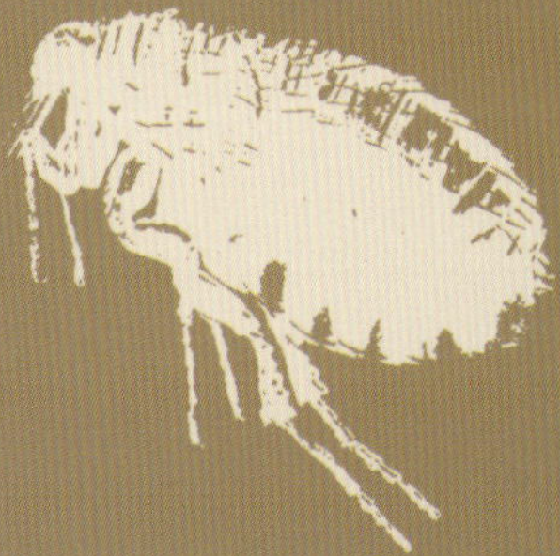

Adult fleas are blood-sucking wingless insects of the order *Siphonaptera*. The word *Siphonaptera* is derived from two words; *siphon* (tube) and *aptera* (wingless). Several different species of fleas are important to domestic animals and most flea species are not host specific.

Perhaps the most complex issue faced by those in the veterinary field is educating the caregiver (client) regarding the difference between treating a flea infestation and the more difficult task of preventing unseen fleas from causing itching in an allergic pet.

Important species of fleas	
Ctenocephalides spp.	The most medically important species. *C. felis felis* causes more than 92 % of dog infestations and 97 % of cat infestations.
Echidnophaga gallinacea	Also known as the sticktight flea of poultry. It can cause infestations in pets in warm climates.
Pulex irritans	It is the human flea and very important as a vector for *Yersinia pestis* (plague). It can also infest dogs and cats.
Spilopsyllus cuniculi	Also known as the rabbit flea, it can also infest cats or dogs, with a predilection for the pinnal or periauricular areas.
Tunga penetrans	It penetrates the epidermis of the host (burrowing flea) and can cause significant morbidity. Once indigenous to regions of Central America, Caribbean and West Indies, it has now spread to Africa, India, Pakistan and South America.

2 General flea anatomy

Main features of flea anatomy [Fig. 1] are as follows:

- Small (1.4–4.0 mm) body of medium-to-dark brown color.
- Like all insects, they have six legs and three body segments.
- The body is laterally compressed and the division of body segments is not readily apparent.
- Powerful legs end in curved claws. The third pair of legs is prominently enlarged.
- Body shape and leg structure facilitate movement on the host and jumping.
- The head of the flea consists of antennae, eyes, combs and mouthparts that are very well adapted for obtaining a blood meal, which is a critical component of the life cycle.

a

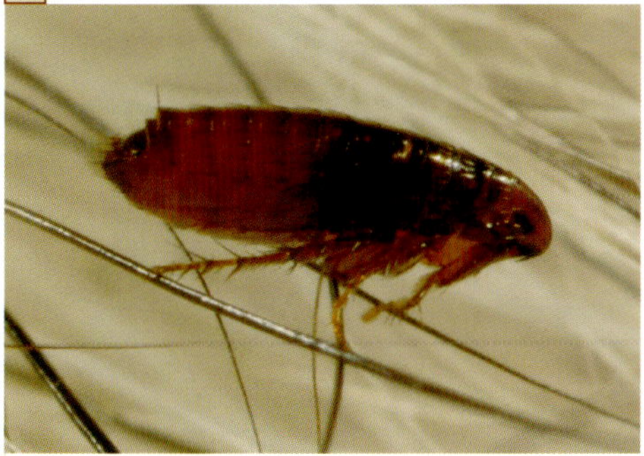

b

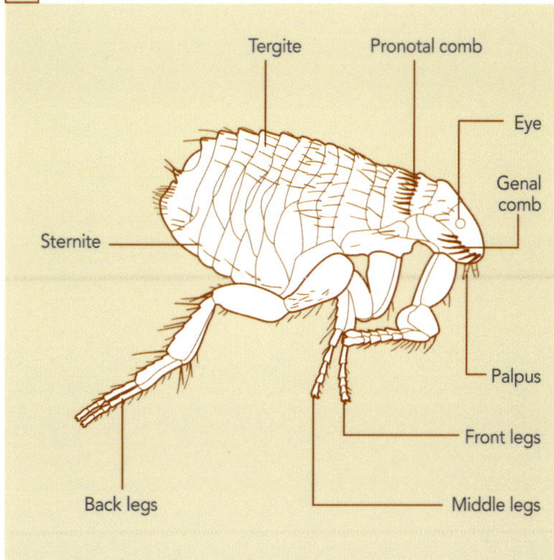

Figure 1. (a) Adult flea of typical color and morphology. This flea is actually on an opossum, which are common sources of fleas that can infest cats and dogs. Image courtesy of Dr. L. Buss and UF/AFIS. (b) Diagram of flea anatomy.

Flea life cycle

Although finding adult fleas on a pet is often the primary reason clients seek flea control options, the complex life cycle of the flea means that once an adult flea is noted, resolution of the problem may not be achievable for three months or more. If a pet is flea allergic, the problem is even more complex.

Refer to *Control measures* section for more specific information.

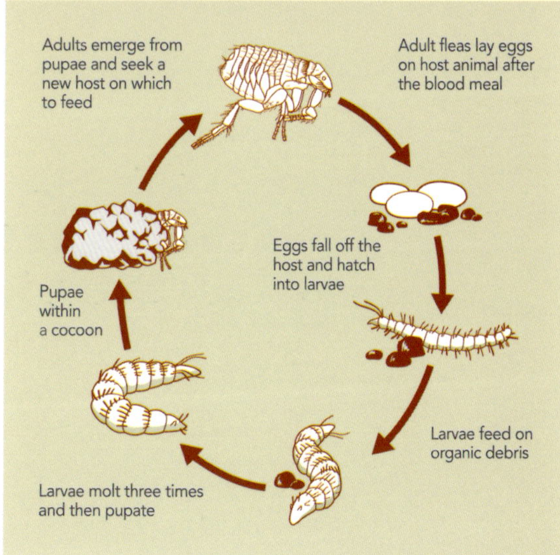

Figure 2. Life cycle of fleas.

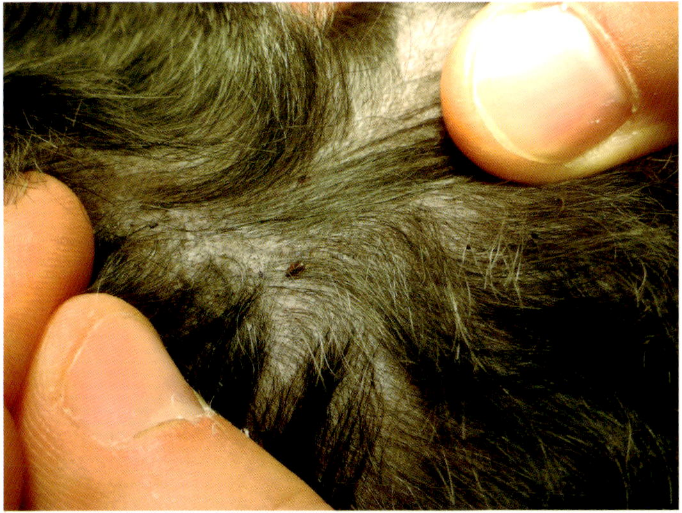

Figure 3. Adult flea and small dark specks of flea feces on a dog.

Finding adult fleas or flea feces often triggers initiation of a flea control program but a proactive preventative plan is preferable.

On-host component of life cycle

Adult fleas and the "blood meal"

Adult fleas spend their entire life either on a host or other contact animals, unless itching or grooming by the host results in dislocation [Fig. 4]. The host provides both protection and food (blood).

Importantly, it is the adult flea's blood meal that results in the vast majority of pathology associated with fleas.

Refer to *Pathology associated with fleas* section for more specific information.

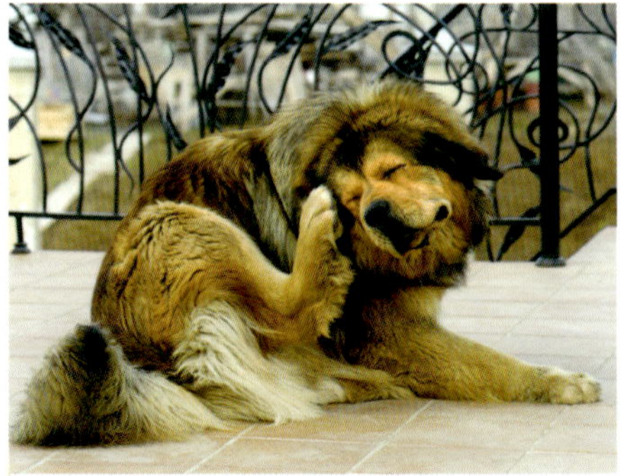

Figure 4. Adult fleas spend their entire life on a host. Image by Neonci/shutterstock.com.

The biology, development and life cycle of *Ctenocephalides felis felis* have been studied in detail and the details discussed here may not apply to other flea species.

Studies show that once fleas are on a host, feeding begins within seconds to minutes and quantifiable amounts of blood are consumed within 5 minutes.

During this feeding action, fleas can cause disease by:

- Mechanically irritating the skin.
- Exposing the host to their saliva.
- Introducing important pathogenic factors.

In association with feeding, fleas excrete incompletely digested blood, which quickly dries into black-to-reddish-black pellets or tubular coils, also known as "flea dirt" [Figs. 5 and 6].

This excrement, after falling into the environment, serves as an important source of food for the larval/nymph life stage.

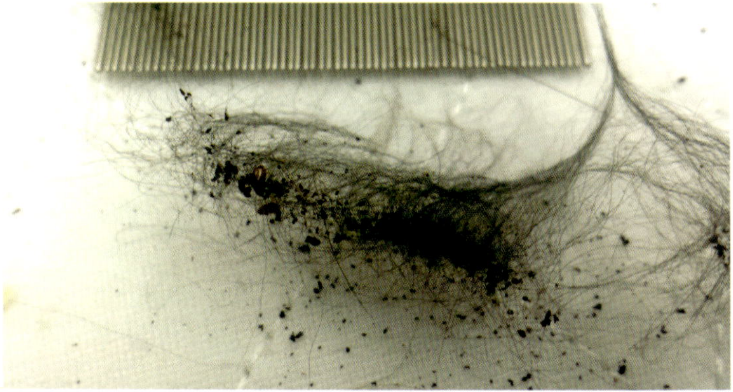

Figure 5. A fine toothed "flea comb" is a convenient mean of finding fleas and flea feces. It is not effective enough to prevent flea infestation or flea-bite induced itching. Image courtesy of A. Foxworth.

The average amount of blood consumed per day by a female cat flea is approximately 15 times its body weight.

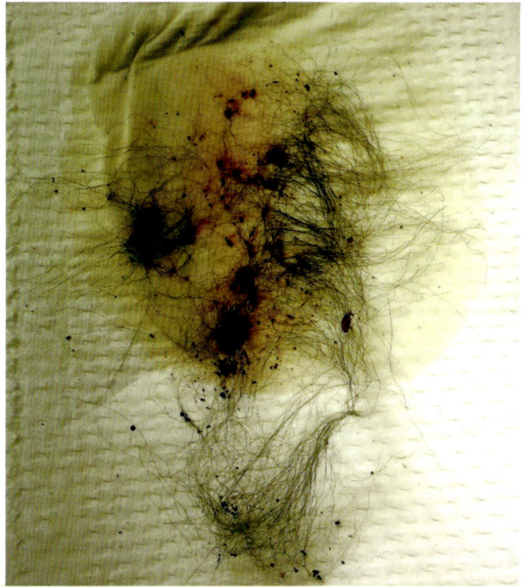

Figure 6. Rubbing a small amount of water into what appears to be dark dirt reveals a red-to-reddish-brown-color indicating that flea dirt is actually flea feces, which consist mostly of digested dried blood. Note the presence of an adult flea in the adjacent strands of hair.

Mating and egg production

A blood meal must occur before fleas initiate the next step of their life cycle: mating. Mating occurs within 8-24 hours of feeding and females begin producing eggs within 24-36 hours.

The eggs, which are not sticky, are laid while the flea is on the host and then drop into the surrounding environment. It is not uncommon for a single female flea to produce 1,300 eggs within 50 days. At her peak, female flea produces up to 40-50 eggs per day. Egg production can occur for more than 100 days, albeit at a gradually declining rate.

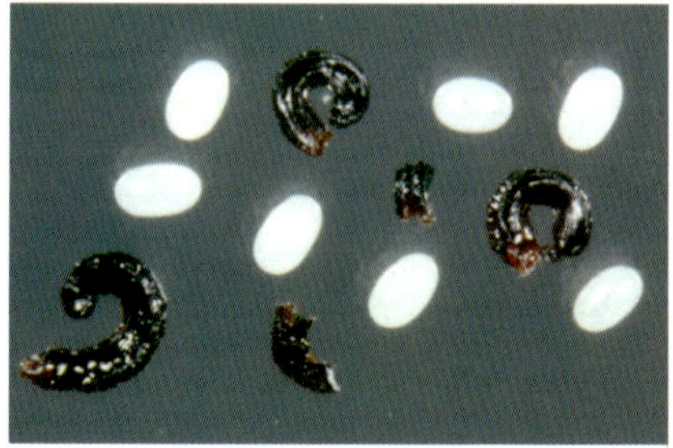

Figure 7. Small, white flea eggs are interspersed between black to slightly red/ brown tubular coils of flea feces (digested dried blood from the host). Flea larvae ingest the flea feces as a source of nutrition. Image courtesy of J. Castner and UF/AFIS.

Environmental component of the life cycle

Complete metamorphosis in the environment completes the remainder of the flea's life cycle. It is very important to realize that the general environment/climate in which a host lives can be considerably different than the microclimate/environment into which the eggs fall and the larvae migrate and develop.

A general climate with temperatures between 20-30 °C and a relative humidity between 60-70 % are ideal for fleas.

Relative humidity is more critical than temperature for survival, except at temperature extremes (below 8 °C or above 35 °C).

Favorable microclimates, such as protected areas around the foundation of a home, or other structures, such as a shed or dog house can offer protection from otherwise harsh environmental conditions.

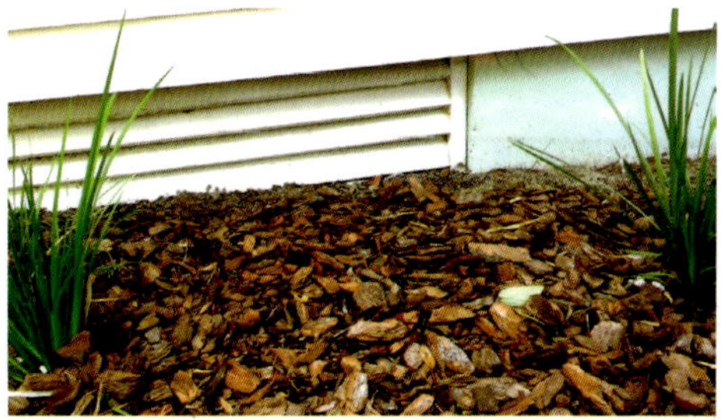

Figure 8. Areas near foundations and vents can provide a safe haven for stray animals and the flea life cycle during inhospitable weather conditions.

Flea eggs in the environment are difficult to see without magnification. They are quite small (0.5 mm), white and oval. Depending on environmental conditions (temperature and humidity), the eggs typically hatch within 1-10 days. Temperatures below 0 °C for 24-36 consecutive hours are lethal to most eggs but protected microclimates, such as within a burrow or near a structure, can offer protection against harsh weather.

The newly hatched larvae are first white like eggs, then become darker in color when they eat the "flea dirt" in the environment [Fig. 9]. They may also feed on other organic debris and flea eggs.

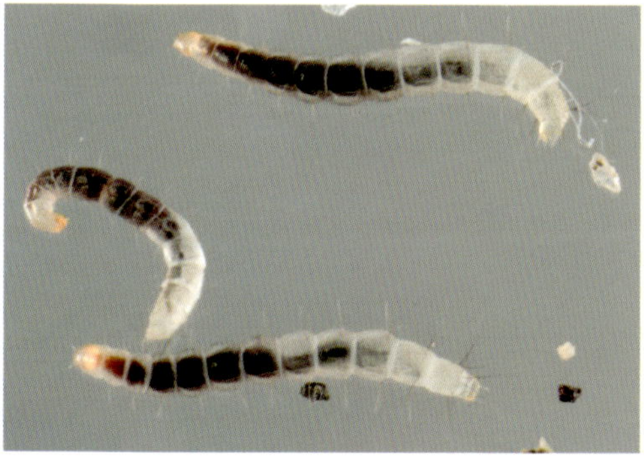

Figure 9. Partially translucent flea larvae are initially white in color but take on the color of their main food source, flea feces, which consist of partially digested blood. Image courtesy of Dr. L. Buss and UF/AFIS.

The larvae are negatively phototactic and positively geotropic, avoiding light and moving deep into their environment. By doing so, they may live in a relatively "protected environment":

- Indoors: deep in carpets, cracks in wood floors, molding inside the home, etc.
- Outdoors: under the soil surface or organic debris.

These protected microenvironments often have a microclimate which may be more conducive to larval survival than the general climate/environment.

Favorable environments/microclimates are often overlooked during a flea control program, leading to frustration and incorrect assumptions regarding efficacy of flea control programs as well as potential misperceptions regarding the development of insecticide resistance among flea populations.

Typically, less than 25 % of larvae survive. Within 5-10 days of hatching, and under ideal conditions, two molts are completed; the third larval instar produces a cocoon [Fig. 10] and pupates.

Pupae are more resistant to environmental stress and the cocoon offers some additional protection. Adult fleas can emerge in as early as 5 days but it can be delayed for up to 140 days.

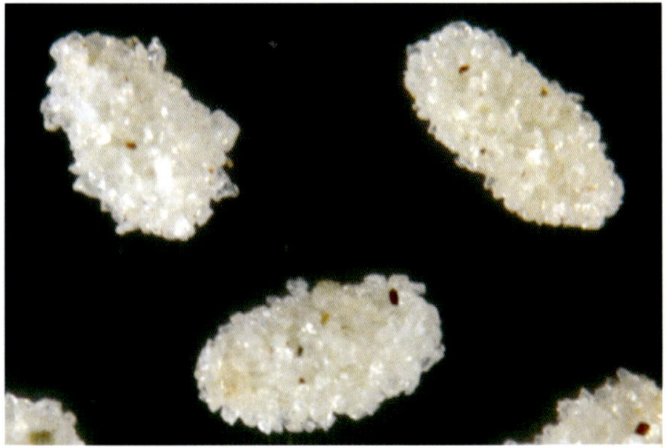

Figure 10. Cocoon stage of the flea cycle with attached debris from the environment. This stage is particularly resistant to insecticides and environmental stress. Image courtesy of J. Castner and UF/AFIS.

Delayed emergence can result in hundreds of "pre-emerged" adults which lie in wait until appropriately stimulated [Fig. 11]. Vibrations and abrupt changes in light intensity, mimicking the passing of a potential host, are stimuli that can cause adults to emerge.

When the stimulus occurs, such as after humans and pets have been absent from the environment for a period of time, a "synchronized emergence" of adult fleas can give the appearance of a "flea explosion". The sudden appearance of many adult fleas often results in frantic phone calls from clients after they return from a vacation.

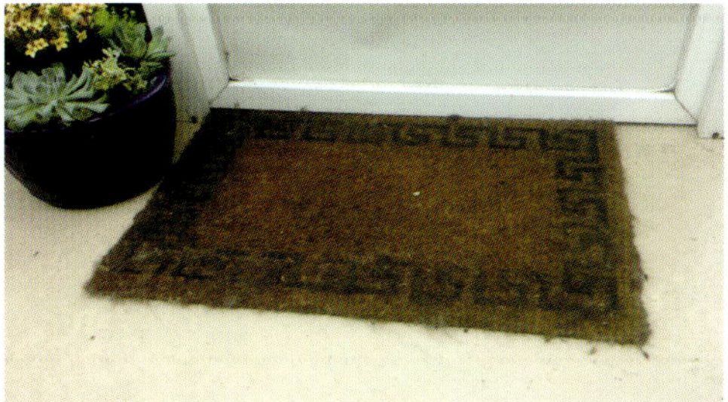

Figure 11. "Pre-emerged" fleas can lie dormant indoors in areas such as carpet or outdoors in a doormat or mulch for weeks or months until stimulated by a potential nearby host.

Additions or alterations in flea treatment protocols for the environment and host may be necessary. The regular use of appropriate preventative measures can prevent this all too common problem.

It is particularly common for an almost imperceptible number of fleas to cause itching in flea-allergic pets.

Although more information regarding flea control follows this section, it is important to realize that because of the "pupated pre-emerged fleas", periodic repeat treatments with an adulticidal insecticide in the environment will likely be necessary for some time as these fleas are stimulated to leave their cocoon and seek a host.

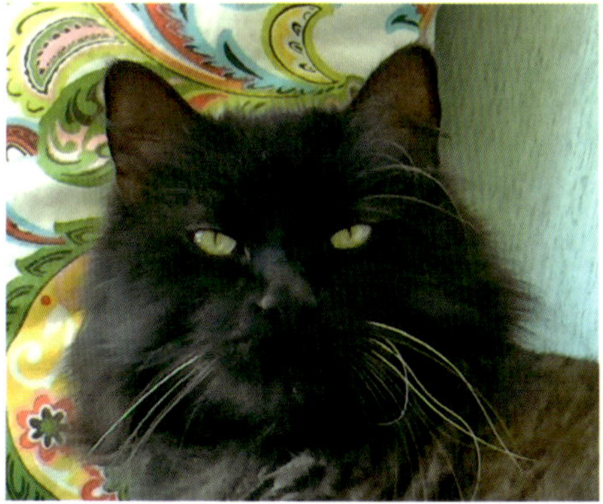

Figure 12. With regular application of flea products, this indoor/outdoor cat enjoys life without flea infestation.
Image courtesy of M. Gram.

Flea-allergic pets can itch due to flea bites in households without any perceived flea infestation. This problem can be difficult for many pet owners and even veterinarians to understand and accept.

In these situations, the adult flea numbers are so low that they are not seen on pets or humans in the environment. If untreated, an unrecognized flea population may expand to significant levels resulting in many pupae and pre-emerged fleas in the environment.

Steps to planning a flea control program

- **Step 1** – Identify the goals
- **Step 2** – Determine and prioritize the attributes of potential products

In clinical veterinary practice, an important first step in planning a flea control program is to identify and articulate the goals of flea control.
Second is to determine and prioritize the attributes of various flea control products or programs. For example:

- The flea control goals involving a non flea-allergic pet can be different than the goals for a flea-allergic pet.
- Or, different flea products may be chosen if a pet is eating a hypoallergenic diet and must avoid flavored oral products.
- Or, if a pet is bathed or swims frequently it would likely benefit from a systemically-acting product or one that replenishes itself.

Flea-allergic pets can itch due to flea bites in without any perceived flea infestation.

- The goals for the non-allergic pet are easier to achieve and can be accomplished much more rapidly.
- The individual attributes of specific products or programs, such as speed of kill or repellency, are typically less important in the long term for the non-allergic pet.
- If, however, a pet is allergic to fleas, constant vigilance and intense preventative measures should be pursued.

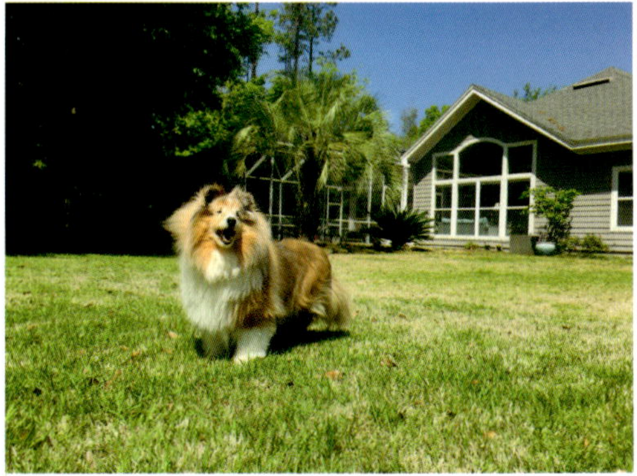

Figure 13. In most climates without a heavy flea burden, the regular use of one of the newer types of flea product will provide adequate flea control and prevent excessive itching due to flea bites for most non flea-allergic pets. Image courtesy of Dr. J. Shmalberg's integrative medicine service at the University of Florida, US.

For basic flea control needs of a non-allergic pet, a single product is often sufficient provided it is one of the newer products that have been developed in the past 20-25 years.

Various formulations exist and the newer products are available as orals, topicals and collars. Previous insecticidal products often were not nearly as effective and/or had a lower margin of safety. Some of the active ingredients in these products have been repackaged to mimic the appearance of the more effective products and offered for sale at a lower cost.

If these products are used, it is not uncommon for fleas to complete their life cycle and lead to an unexpected flea problem. This is common in warmer and relatively humid climates. In these climates, a flea-allergic pet has additional challenges.

The use of a "double down" flea control program may be advisable in some situations.

Refer to *Control measures* section for more specific information (pages 39-41).

Once adult fleas are noted on a pet, clients must be prepared for the reality that 3-6 months of intensive flea control measures may be necessary before they should expect to "not see any fleas". Even if general improvement can be expected much sooner than this, occasional adult fleas may be occasionally noted.

This unfortunate phenomenon is due to pre-emerged fleas [see Fig. 13] lying in wait within a cocoon, where they may be protected from recent "catch-up" flea control measures. They then emerge days to weeks after the environmental treatment and seek a blood meal.

Depending on the number of fleas emerging, repellant efficacy, and the speed of kill of the products used on the host, adult fleas will be present. They may not die quickly and thus seek a host in order to obtain their important blood meal and induce pruritus. It is particularly common for an almost imperceptible number of fleas to cause itching in flea-allergic pets [Figs. 14 and 15].

In the flea-allergic patient, the symptoms of itching can be quite disturbing while adult fleas may actually never be seen.

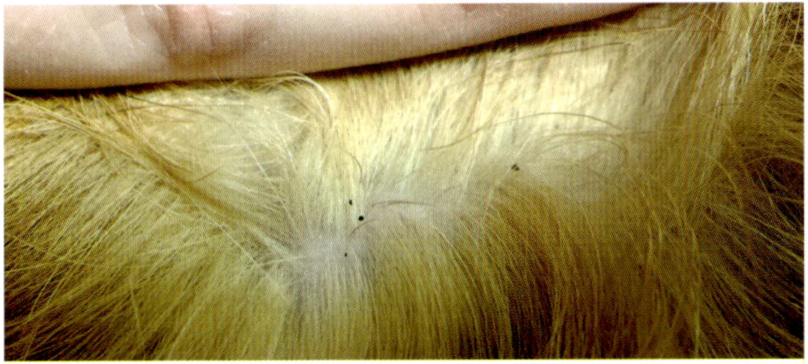

Figure 14. It may be easier to find small dark specks of flea dirt (flea feces) than the actual adult fleas on some pets.

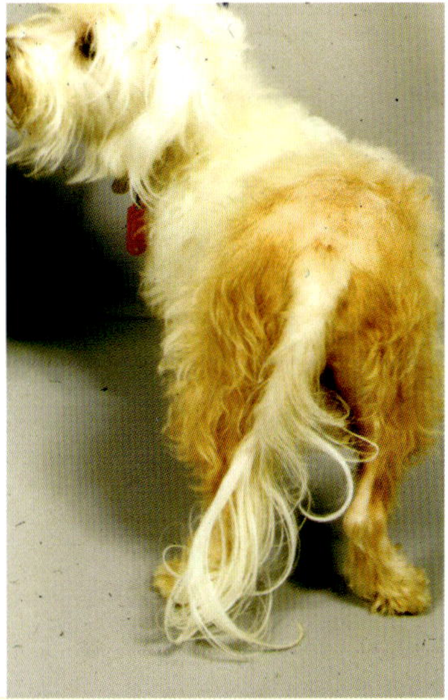

Figure 15. Adult fleas were not seen on this patient. Hair loss and salivary staining associated with chewing and licking of the rump and thigh region is a classic feature of flea allergy dermatitis (FAD). Intradermal allergy testing demonstrated a very strong reaction to fleas. This dog also suffered from environmental allergies which responded well to allergen-specific immunotherapy injections.

Prioritizing aspects of flea control products/programs

Different flea control programs may include the need for any of the following traits (see next page). The relative priority of these attributes may change based on individual circumstances and other animal species that share the same environment.

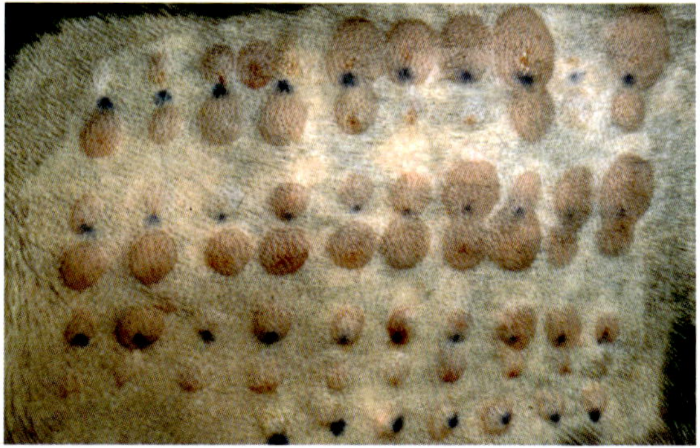

Figure 16. Intradermal allergy test on a dog revealing reactions to fleas as well as many environmental allergens.

Prioritizing attributes of flea control products

- Presence of cats with close contact to treated dogs: some dog products, notably repellants before they have dried, can be lethal to cats.
- Pet/client preference: oral, topical, collar, ease of use, etc.
- Frequency of application: many products are labeled for being applied once a month, but some have extended periods of efficacy.
- Concurrent heartworm prevention: the use of products with multiple purposes may improve compliance.
- Price: if a pet has other medical issues requiring therapy (arthritis, special dietary needs), the costs of managing multiple issues can be an important factor.
- Empirical scabies mite treatment: some flea-allergic dogs are so pruritic that scabies mite infestation is an important differential diagnosis.

Most instances of suspected resistance are actually due to a less-than-instantaneous speed of kill or recently emerged fleas that were previously in the protected pupal stage. These situations are very common in areas with a high flea burden.

Killing adult fleas effectively can significantly reduce, if not totally eliminate, a flea infestation. For flea allergy dermatitis (FAD) patients, killing adult fleas is not enough because many products take 48 hours to kill.

- Concurrent tick control.
- Persistent efficacy: flea-allergic pets benefit from consistent elimination of adult fleas from the household and rapid kill of any adult fleas that try to infest.
- Concurrent intestinal and other parasite control.
- Concurrent hypoallergenic dietary trial: take into account that it would be compromised by any flavored oral products.
- Efficacy regarding frequent bathing or swimming: oral or topical products acting systemically may be desirable.
- Potential insecticide resistance or perceived resistance within the local flea population: first make sure that the treatment is being used correctly, because incorrect treatment use is more common than flea resistance.

Some dog products, especially repellants, can be lethal to cats.

The finding of several fleas on a pet within a few weeks of initiating a flea control program should actually be expected as adult fleas develop from pre-existing pupae, and should not be interpreted to mean that a flea control product or program is failing.

Determining the goals of a flea control program

By the time adult fleas are noted on a pet, their life cycle is likely entrenched in the environment. Depending on the number of pre-emerged fleas present, even a properly executed flea control program will require several weeks to months until full success can be achieved.

Fleas may actually be expected for a few months, albeit in declining numbers. For the flea-allergic pet, unseen fleas contribute to itching for a considerably longer period of time before the flea life cycle is completely disrupted.

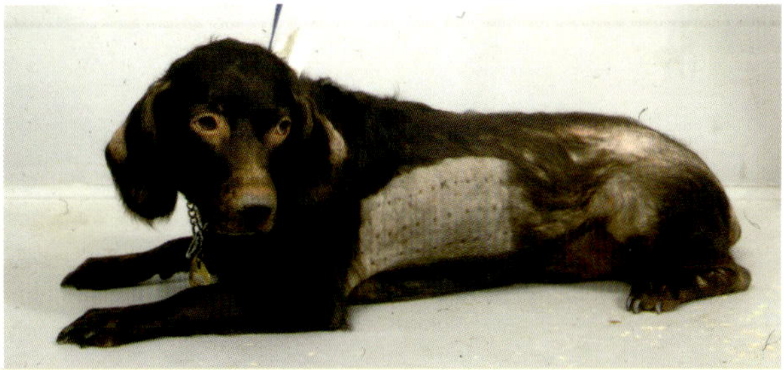

Figure 17. This patient exhibited symptoms of dermatitis and otitis due to flea allergies and atopic dermatitis. Both flea control measures and allergen-specific immunotherapy were necessary to control the symptoms.

Articulating the needs of a household with regards to the goals of flea control program helps set expectations and provides a framework for education.

The goals may include the following: (1) significantly reducing the number of fleas seen on a pet; (2) eliminating fleas from being seen on a pet; (3) preventing fleas from causing pruritus or dermatitis; and (4) eliminating fleas in the environment.

Goal 1: significantly reducing the number of fleas seen on a pet

This is one of the goals easier to achieve, however, it does require persistence and patience.

As previously discussed, regular use of one of the somewhat recently developed products should be effective at preventing an obvious flea infestation. If fleas are noted while following this protocol, it is typically due to a lapse or even slight delay in the frequency of administration.

Most commonly, these seen fleas are not actually resistant to the products used, but were in the life cycle stage most resistant to treatment during environmental control measures, i.e. the pupae within a cocoon. They then emerged from the pupae and jumped onto a pet.

Depending on the adulticidal or repellant control measures used on the pet, the fleas may not quickly die or be adequately repelled. These surviving fleas serve as a reminder that the easiest means of preventing flea infestations is consistent and regular application of products that break the flea life cycle and prevent fleas from entering the pupal stage of the life cycle. Missing an application by even a few days can be associated with a much slower speed of kill and the finding of adult fleas.

If adult fleas are noted within a few weeks of starting or restarting a flea control program, it is very important to also investigate the possibility of an overlooked or undertreated area. These "point source" areas are typically conducive to the flea life cycle but can be difficult to treat.

"Point source" is a term referring to an often relatively small area conducive to the flea life cycle that serves as a source of continual flea exposure (see Figs. 8, 11, 18, 19, 22).

Areas inside the home include under furniture, pet bedding, human bedding or cat trees [Fig. 18], which can be easily overlooked when treating the environment.

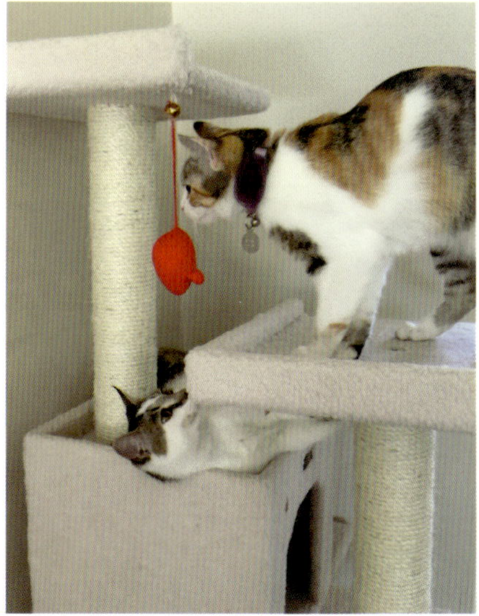

Figure 18. Depending on the extent of a flea infestation, using environmental control measures in the home may be necessary and should include treating areas favorable to the flea life cycle, including cat trees, carpeted areas and pet bedding. Image courtesy of M. Gram.

Point source areas outside the home may include outdoor carpeting, doormats, corners of planting beds, under shrubbery, porches [Fig. 19] and areas where untreated wild or domestic animals rest are also common "point sources".

In many geographic regions, feral cats or dogs and various small wild mammals can complicate an already challenging situation.

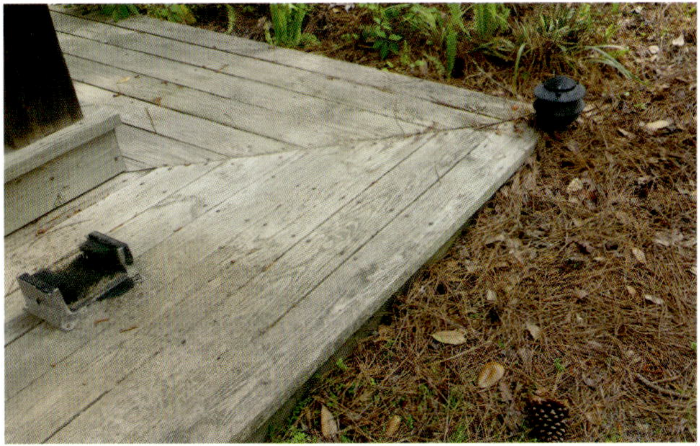

Figure 19. The cracks between the boards on this shaded wooden deck provide an excellent area in which flea eggs may fall through and complete their life cycle.

Goal 2: eliminating fleas from being seen on a pet

This is the expected goal that most clients have regarding the use of flea control products. It is a reasonable goal that is eventually possible in most, but not all, situations. If a patient is allergic to fleas, this goal may still not be enough to prevent itching and dermatitis.

Unseen adult fleas may bite, die and fall off or be ingested before ever being seen. With chronic strict environmental control measures and a very good repellant or fast killing adulticidal product, this goal can be achieved.

The steps necessary to reach this goal depend on the flea burden within the home as well as outside. Favorable outdoor climates and environment can be a barrier to success. Total elimination of seeing adult fleas may not be possible if an animal has access to the outside environment due to unseen untreated animals that can carry fleas.

Refer to section above with regards to stray/feral outdoor animals and "point sources".

In flea-allergic pets, the goal of simply not seeing fleas may still not be enough to prevent itching and dermatitis.

The use of adulticidal flea products and appropriate insect growth regulators in the outdoor environment can help prevent a flea population from becoming established but does not guarantee that an occasional "opportunistic flea" will not make its way into the environment.

Depending on the speed of kill or repellency of products used on a pet, adult fleas may actually be seen even when good flea control is being utilized. Appropriate use of the right product should prevent these rare fleas from being able to complete their life cycle.

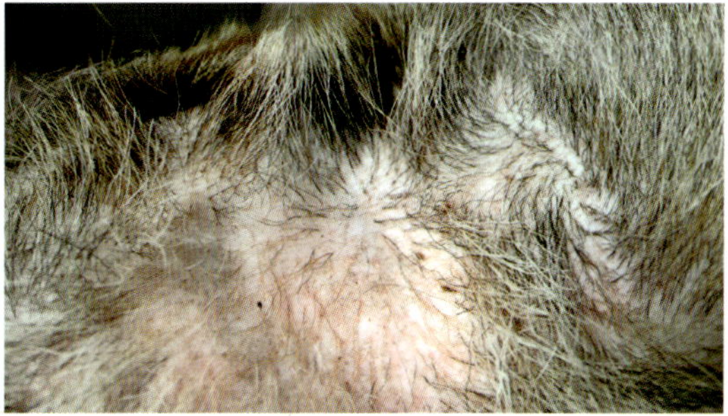

Figure 20. The major symptom of this patient was itching but the owner had not noticed any fleas. Although the "rump" and caudal thighs are often preferred areas for fleas, they may be more easily visualized on the abdomen in some patients. Image courtesy of A. Beaver.

Goal 3: preventing fleas from causing pruritus or dermatitis

For the vast majority of pets, achieving the first two goals would result in the accomplishment of this goal. However, for the flea-allergic pet, that is NOT TRUE.

In these circumstances, an exceptionally low number of fleas are present but fleas are not seen in the environment or on other pets and do not feed on humans sharing the household. Even humans with "sensitive skin" may never have evidence of flea bites. The following KEY POINTS are important for thorough client education.

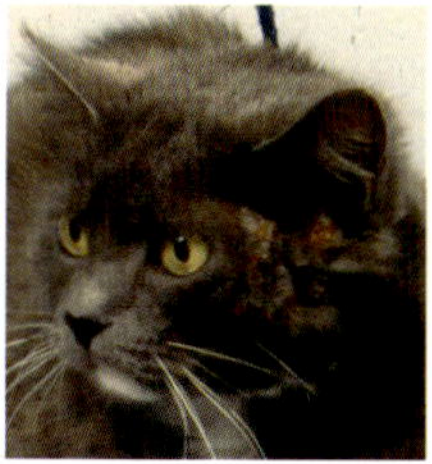

Figure 21. While most cats with fleas or suffering from flea allergy will lick or chew their dorsum or abdomen, some will scratch intently at their neck or face. Environmental allergies or food allergies may cause identical symptoms.

Using the analogy of mosquitoes and their preference for biting certain humans and the individual's sensitivity to those bites can be a useful educational tool while discussing important aspects of a flea control program with pet owners.

KEY POINTS for client education

In the flea-allergic patient, the symptom of itching can be quite notable even when adult fleas are not seen.

When prompted, many clients report that their pet's itching increases in the days preceding the scheduled reapplication of product.

Flea-allergic patients often harbor fewer fleas than non-flea allergic pets in the same environment, making it less likely to see fleas when they are present.

Although killing adult fleas can significantly reduce a flea infestation, this alone may not be adequate because many products require 48 hours to kill most of the adult fleas. This delayed kill is especially noted 1-14 days BEFORE the product is due to be reapplied. These not-yet-dead fleas may feed several times over a period of many hours before they die. The allergic pet will chew and scratch after being bitten and often ingest or dislodge the fleas, further decreasing the likelihood that they will be seen.

III As previously discussed, once adult fleas are noted, 3-6 months of highly effective treatment may be required before one can expect to "not see any fleas." If a pet is flea allergic or a significant environmental infestation is present, additional flea control measures should be pursued. Eliminating all (or nearly all) fleas and life stages in the environment will eventually be achieved and no fleas will be biting an allergic pet.

Ongoing flea control is still very important because animals can be reinfested with exposure to other pets or from outdoor flea populations maintained on wild animals. [Fig. 22].

IV The use of a "double down" protocol has proven valuable for some animals; however, new effective systemic treatments are offering an alternative option for adult flea control in allergic animals. This protocol typically uses two different products with different active

ingredients and attributes: one product is used at the beginning of the month and another product is used in the middle of the month. While some "monthly" flea products are labeled for use more than once a month, some are not and doing so could violate label instructions and laws.

The use of a "double down" flea control protocol can be very helpful in managing the flea allergic pet or a pet with various parasite control needs.

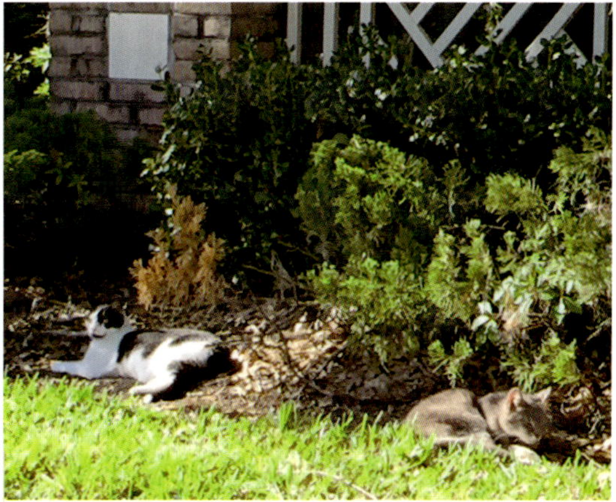

Figure 22. Feral or wild animals may be undetected and visit the yards and porches of homes. These animals are common sources of flea infestations and may harbor diseases that fleas can transmit. Image courtesy of M. Gram.

If using "double down" flea control, it is important to know the active ingredients of products in order to avoid using different brand names but similar active ingredients.

The use of products with different active ingredients allows the following benefits.

- For virtually all products, the speed of kill is typically faster for the first 2 weeks after a product is applied. The label instructions on some products may not allow more frequent application and the use of a different product with different active ingredients can overcome this issue. Many studies report the percentage of fleas killed 28 days after product application whereas many months are actually 31 days long. These few extra days can be very important when a patient is flea allergic.
- Different products may have different attributes that are desirable in certain situations.

Refer to *Prioritizing aspects of flea control products/programs* for more specific information (pages 28 and 29).

Goal 4: eliminating fleas in the environment

The absolute elimination of fleas in the environment is only possible under some conditions over a period of many months. The efficacy of most "host-applied treatments" is so high that, given enough time, the life cycle of the flea can be interrupted.

Long-term environmental flea control may not be necessary in many situations. Environmental flea control measures should be practiced if a pet is flea allergic, or exposed to an environment or climate with a history of a high flea burden, or visited by untreated wild or domestic animals.

These measures typically utilize a product containing two different ingredients: one product that will kill adult fleas and another that will interrupt their life cycle, such as an insect growth regulator (IGR), which prevents the pupation of the flea larvae.

5 Pathology associated with fleas

Flea saliva itself can cause irritation or allergies. During feeding, fleas can consume large volumes of blood and serve as vectors for many disease-causing organisms [Fig. 23].

The scope of this publication does not include how to diagnose and treat disease associated with fleas but rather to raise awareness through education and emphasize the need for flea control.

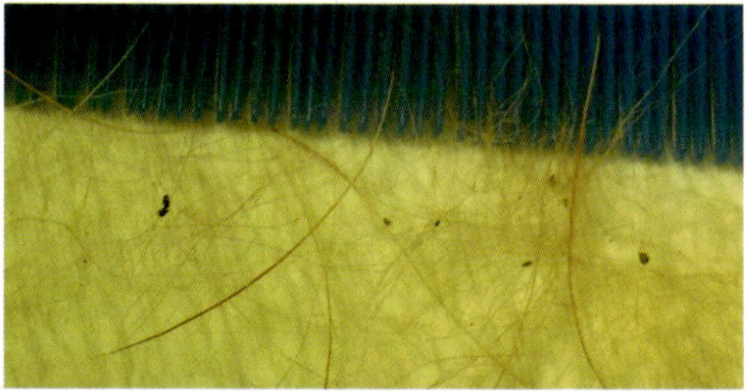

Figure 23. Although close examination, including the use of a flea comb, is an excellent means of monitoring the presence of fleas or flea feces, it is not an effective means of preventing pathology associated with fleas and flea bites. In fact, once adult fleas are noted, they may have already transmitted disease and caused itching or dermatitis.

Anemia

Severe flea infestations and flea feeding can result in life threatening anemia, particularly in young [Fig. 24] or small patients.

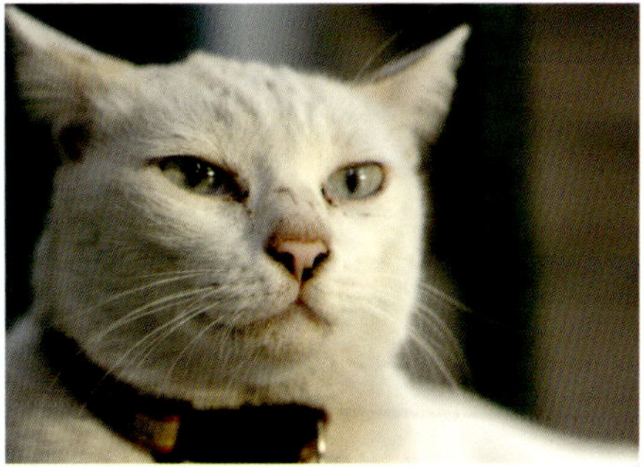

Figure 24. Anemia may be one of the first signs of flea infestation. Note the pale mucous membranes suggesting anemia in this cat.
Image by suradach/shutterstock.com.

Tapeworms

Fleas are the intermediate host for the tapeworm *Dipylidium caninum*, which can affect both dogs and cats. In humans, they are usually self-limiting and typically clear spontaneously within six weeks.

Pruritus

It is a common misconception among clients that in order for fleas to cause pruritus, fleas must be seen either on the affected patient or some other pet or human in the household. Although fleas are often

seen in these situations, as previously discussed, they may not be seen but still cause problems. This pruritus can occur due to several factors [Fig. 25].

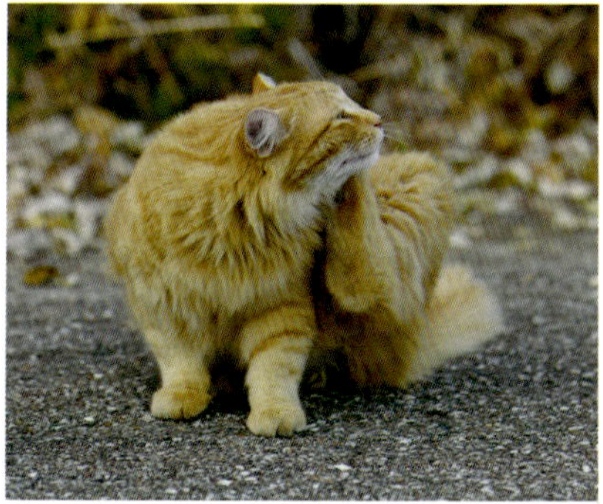

Figure 25. Pruritus may be present even if no fleas have been observed on the pet. Image by Steve Collender/shutterstock.com.

- Obviously, when a flea bites a flea-allergic pet, an allergic inflammatory reaction ensues. The traditional statement that "One flea bite can cause a flea-allergic pet to itch for two weeks" is a useful quote. However, it may not be entirely accurate. Significantly reducing the number of flea-feeding episodes can result in a dramatically lower level of pruritus.
- A complex interaction between flea-feeding induced inflammation and pruritus occurs with a patient that has concomitant atopic dermatitis. A patient with atopic dermatitis often has "sensitive skin" and even minor triggers can induce pruritus. The concept of "summation of effect" and pruritic threshold, along with advances in our understanding of "pruritic pathophysiology" may help explain this phenomenon. An additional complexity includes the use of

a validated pruritus visual analog scale (VAS), which helps differentiate varying degrees of pruritus.

- Infections secondary to flea bites and self-trauma may be pruritic. Repeated use of antibiotics can predispose to these infections becoming resistant. Methicillin-resistant staphylococcal infections are not uncommon.

Dermatitis

The flea bite itself can cause dermatitis alone and lead to secondary infections that may not be pruritic. This is more common in cats than in dogs. The caudal dorsal or "rump" area and neck regions are the more commonly affected areas.

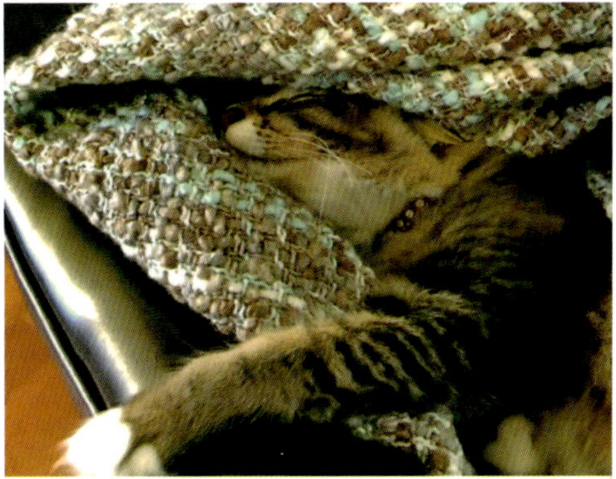

Figure 26. Regular use of flea control products is the most effective means of preventing flea infestations and flea-associated diseases. Image of this healthy cat is courtesy of Dr. Gary Ellison's surgical skills and the University of Florida, US.

Potential flea-transmitted diseases

Fleas can be vectors for *Rickettsia*, *Bartonella*, *Mycoplasma* (hemoplasma) and potentially other organisms of zoonotic significance.

The mechanical action of feeding and some of the contents of flea saliva can cause itching without a true allergic reaction.

6 References

Blagburn BL, Dryden MW. Biology, treatment and control of flea and tick infestations. *Vet. Clin. N. Am.* 2009, 39(6):1173–1200.

Dryden MW. Flea and tick control in the 21st century, challenges and opportunities. *Vet. Dermatol.* 2009, 20, 435–440.

Kramer F, Mencke N. Flea Biology and Control, Springer. 2001, 1-8:1–62.

Miller WH, Griffin CE, Campbell KL. Muller and Kirk's Small Animal Dermatology, 7th edition, Elsevier Inc. 2013, 6:322–329.

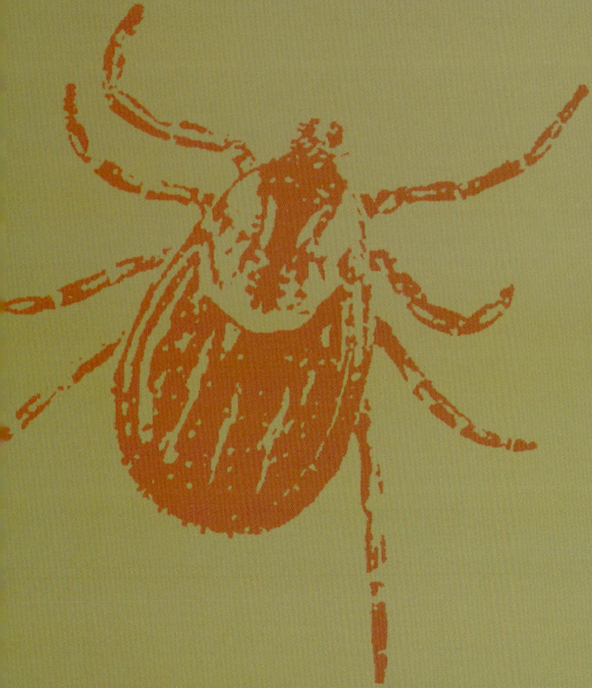

TICKS

Jeanmarie Short
DVM

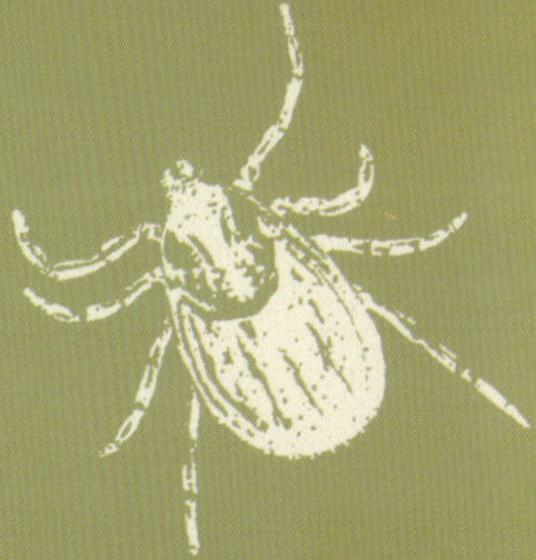

Introduction

Ticks are divided into two types: hard and soft. Hard ticks are so-named because of the shield (scutum) covering the dorsal surface of the tick. Soft ticks do not have this distinctive characteristic. Their differences are also seen in life cycles, lifespan and disease transmission. There are significantly more known species of hard ticks than soft ones. Soft ticks tend to produce fewer eggs and are less parasitic compared to hard ticks.

Soft ticks

- Fewer eggs laid
- Less species

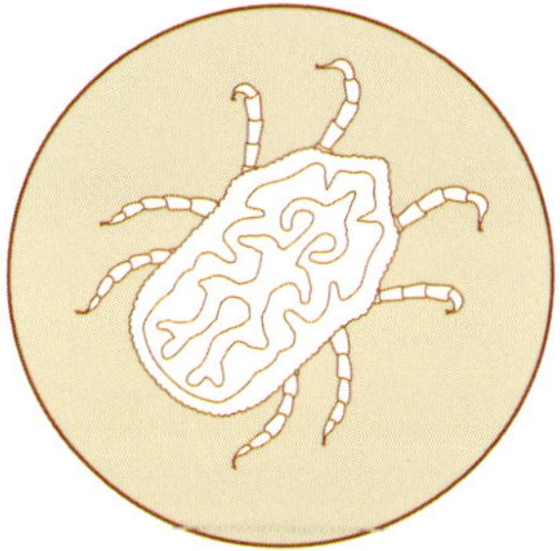

Hard ticks

- Large quantity of eggs laid
- More species

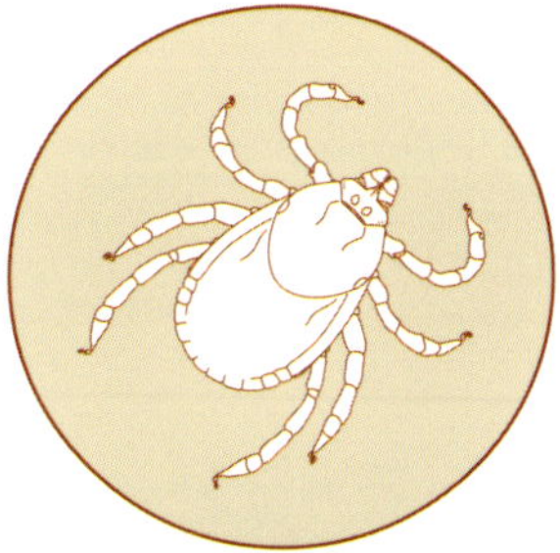

Hard ticks

The differentiating feature in hard ticks is the scutum that covers the male's dorsal body and partially covers the female's [Figs. 1 and 2]. The shorter scutum of the female allows her body to expand during a blood meal.

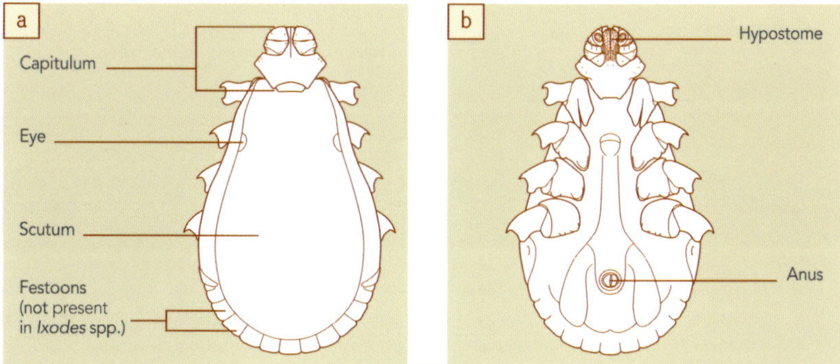

Figure 1. Male hard tick, dorsum (a) and ventrum (b).

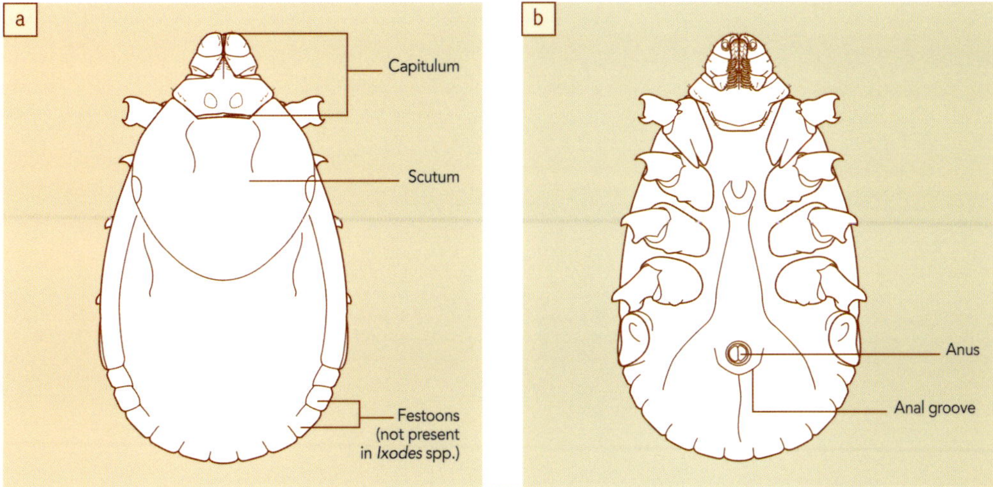

Figure 2. Female hard tick, dorsum (a) and ventrum (b).

Tick feeding

The hypostome – the part of the tick that inserts into the host for a blood meal – is covered by chelicerae. These chelicerae retract slowly during the feeding process, in a breaststroke-like movement, and allow the hypostome to propel deeper into the host. The hypostome itself has unidirectional barb-like projections that are inserted into the host's skin, which help prevent removal.

Tick saliva contains many enzymes and proteins that facilitate the feeding process, such as anesthetic-like substances and blood-clotting inhibitors. Some ticks also release a cement-like compound that help them attach more firmly to the host, making removal more difficult. While ticks are taking a blood meal, any pathogens the tick may be harboring will be passed to the host through the saliva.

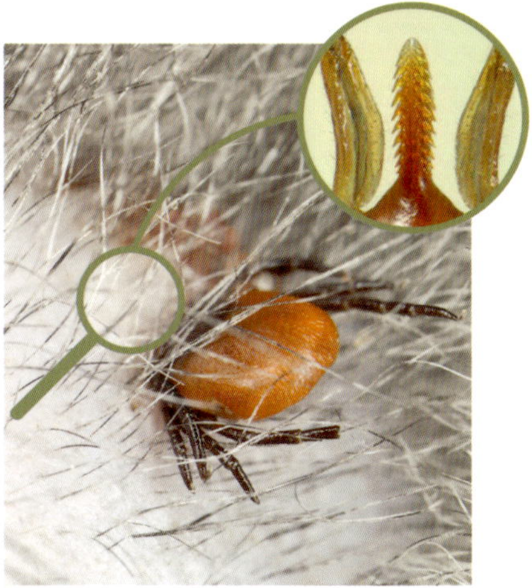

Figure 3. Tick feeding on a cat. Detail of the hypostome, note the unidirectional barbs. Image by Henrik Larsson/shutterstock.com.

Hard tick life cycle

The hard ticks that are covered in this section follow a three-host life cycle [Fig. 4]. Each stage requires a blood meal from a new host before molting. Nymphs take a blood meal from another host and molt to adult stages.

> **For all species, the life cycle is very dependent on environmental temperatures and humidity as well as availability of hosts. Its length varies with genus and species.**

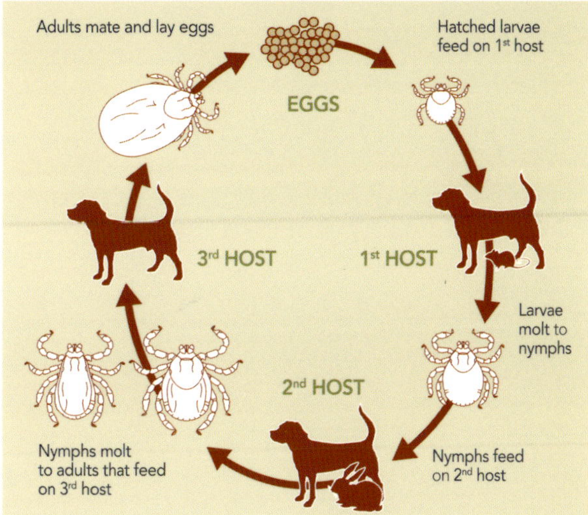

Figure 4. Three-host life cycle.

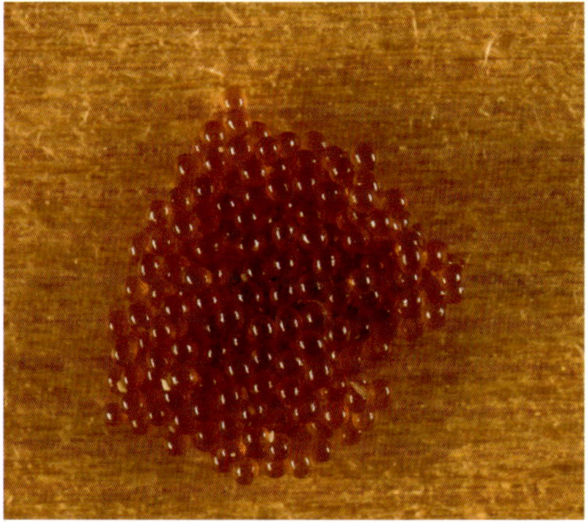

Figure 5. Eggs from a brown dog tick (*Rhipicephalus sanguineus*). Image courtesy of Lyle J. Buss, Entomology and Nematology Department, University of Florida, US.

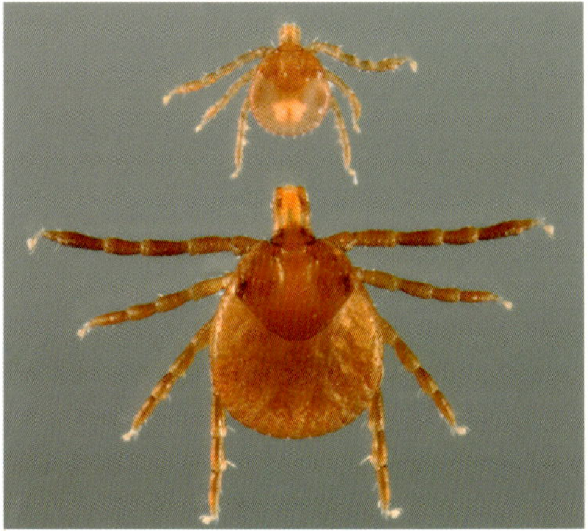

Figure 6. Larva (top) and nymph (bottom) of the lone star tick (*Amblyomma americanum*). Image courtesy of Lyle J. Buss, Entomology and Nematology Department, University of Florida, US.

To facilitate finding a host, ticks climb up vegetation and extend legs. This is called questing [Fig. 7]. As a host passes by, questing ticks are picked up and then move around the host until a feeding site is found.

Questing is a typical behavior of hard ticks.

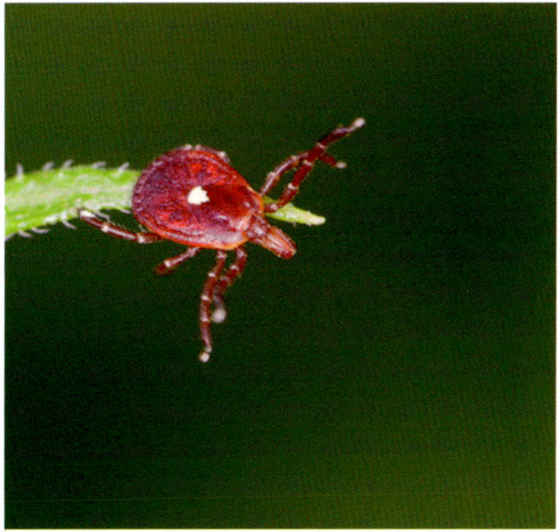

Figure 7. Lone star tick (*Amblyomma americanum*) questing on a blade of grass. Image courtesy of Anthony Zukoff.

Rhipicephalus spp.

Rhipicephalus genus is made up of approximately 79 species. *Rhipicephalus sanguineus*, also known as the brown dog tick, is one of the more recognized in the group.

R. sanguineus can be found throughout the US and worldwide [Table 1].

R. sanguineus can be endophilic, i.e. ecologically associated with humans and their domestic environment, which is a unique feature. These ticks can frequently be found indoors, in carpet and furniture, and climbing walls while seeking a host.

Most of the tick's life (94-97 %) is spent off-host.

Table 1. Common names for *R. sanguineus*.

Name	Area
Brown dog tick	United States, South Africa, Australia
Kennel tick	United Kingdom
Tropical dog tick	South Africa

Dogs are the primary host for all life stages [Table 2, Figs. 8-10] but rarely can be found on other mammals, including humans, because they are opportunistic.

Table 2. Life stages of *R. sanguineus*.

Stage	Dimensions	Aspect	Comments
Larvae	0.5 mm long, 0.4 mm wide	Off-white, light yellow	Feed for 3-10 days; molt 5-15 days; can survive up to 8 months without a meal.
Nymph	1-1.3 mm long, 0.5-0.6 mm wide	Yellow, light brown	Feed 3-11 days; molt 9-47 days; can survive up to 6 months without a meal.
Adult male	2-3 mm long, 1-1.6 mm wide	Flat, reddish brown, tiny pits over dorsum	Can survive up to 19 months without a meal.
Adult female	2-3 mm long, 1-1.6 mm wide	Similar to males except shorter scutum	Feed for 5-21 days; can survive up to 19 months without a meal.
Engorged female	Up to 11.5 mm long, 7.5 mm wide	Gray-green with brown scutum	Oviposition period is 16-18 days, after eggs are laid the female dies.

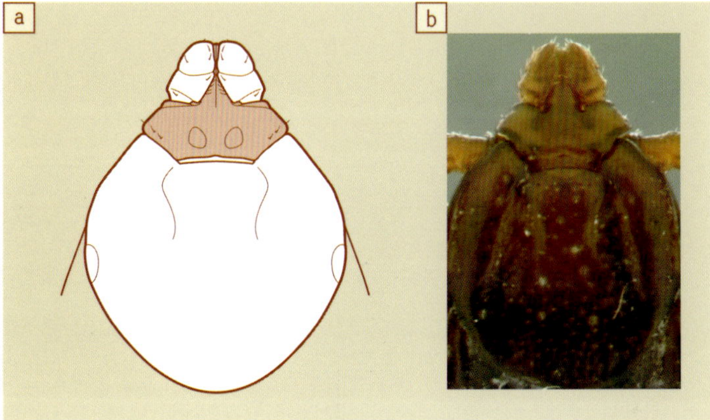

Figure 8. (a) Diagram and (b) photo of the head and scutum of *Rhipicephalus* spp. Highlighted portion indicates hexagonal capituli shape noted in the genus.
Image courtesy of Lyle J. Buss, Entomology and Nematology Department, University of Florida, US.

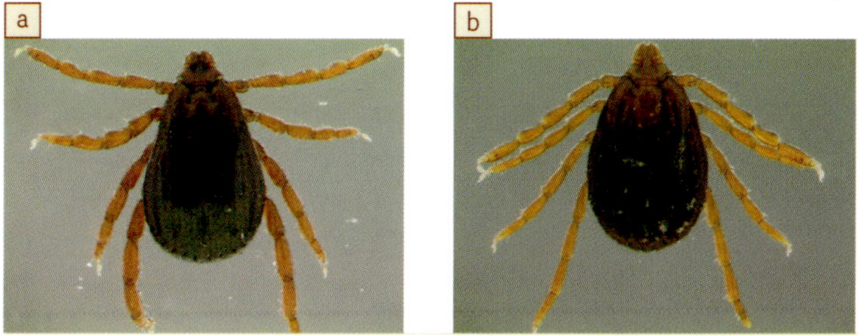

Figure 9. *R. sanguineus.*
(a) Male. (b) Female.
Image courtesy of Lyle J. Buss, Entomology and Nematology Department, University of Florida, US.

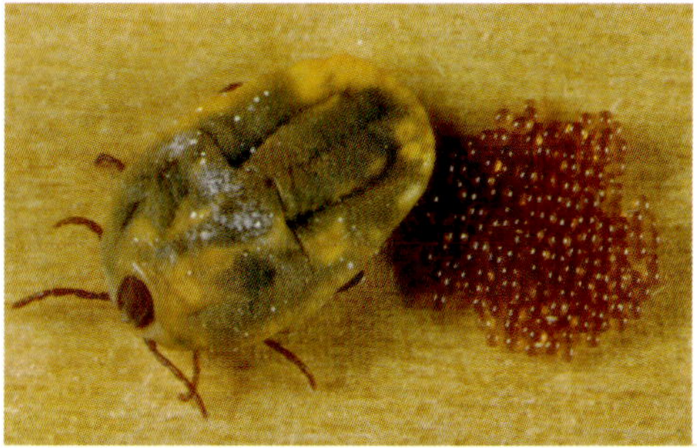

Figure 10. Engorged *R. sanguineus* female and eggs.
Image courtesy of Lyle J. Buss, Entomology and Nematology Department, University of Florida, US.

Amblyomma spp.

Two widespread, common species of the genus *Amblyomma* in the United States include *A. americanum* [lone star tick, Figs. 11-13] and *A. maculatum* [Gulf Coast tick, Figs. 14 and 15].

The lone star tick is most notable due to the white spot on the scutum of the female [Fig. 12].

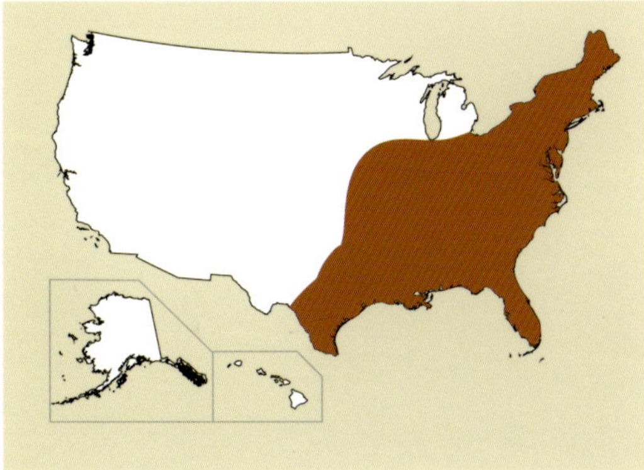

Figure 11. Distribution of lone star tick (*A. americanum*) in the United States.

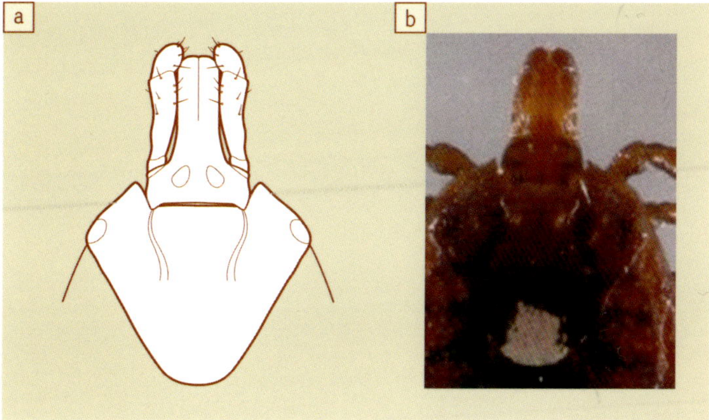

Figure 12. (a) Diagram and (b) photo of the head and scutum of *A. americanum*.
Image courtesy of Lyle J. Buss, Entomology and Nematology Department, University of Florida, US.

Adults of lone star ticks (*A. americanum*) parasitize medium and large mammals (including cattle), and the larvae and nymphs feed on a wide variety of small-to-large mammals and ground-feeding birds, although availability of large mammalian hosts is essential to maintain large populations [Table 3].

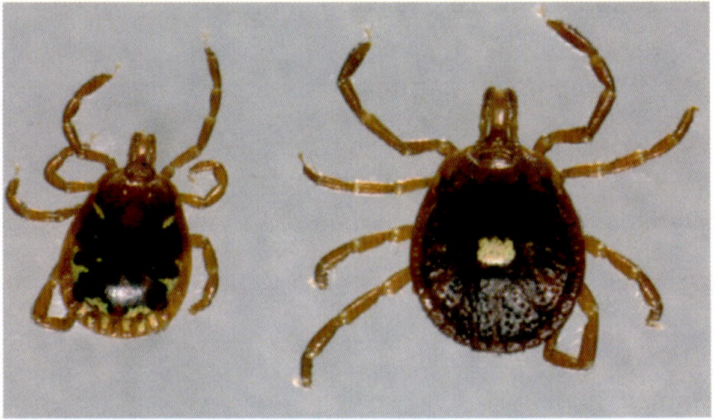

Figure 13. Lone star ticks (*A. americanum*), male (left) and female (right). Image courtesy of by Jerry F. Butler, Entomology and Nematology Department, University of Florida, US.

Table 3. Life stages of *A. americanum.*			
Stage	**Dimensions**	**Aspect**	**Comments**
Larvae	0.5-1 mm long	White to light brown	Feed for 4-9 days; molt in 3-4 weeks; can survive up to 6 months without feeding.
Nymph	1.5-2.5 mm long	Light brown	Feed 3-8 days; molt in 5-6 weeks; can survive up to 6 months without feeding.
Adult male [Fig. 14]	3-4 mm long	Brown with various white streaks/spots on scutum	A blood meal is needed for mating; can survive 8 months to 2 years without feeding.
Adult female [Fig. 14]	3-4 mm long	Brown with white spot on center of scutum	Can survive 8 months to 2 years without feeding.
Engorged female	11 mm long	Gray, yellow	Thousands of eggs may be laid before female dies.

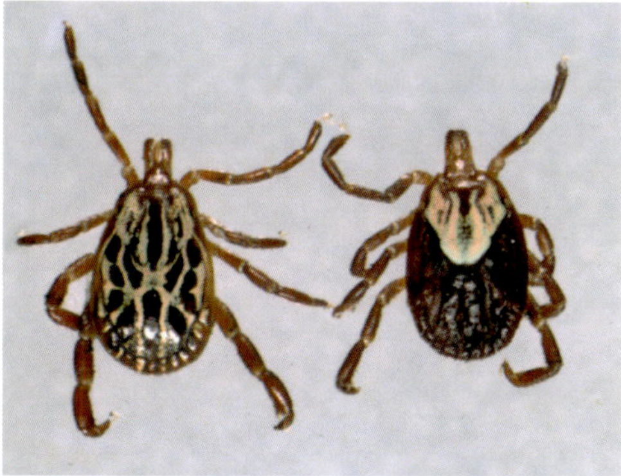

Figure 14. Gulf Coast ticks (*A. maculatum*), male (left) and female (right). Note the ornamental scutum. Image courtesy of by Jerry F. Butler, Entomology and Nematology Department, University of Florida, US.

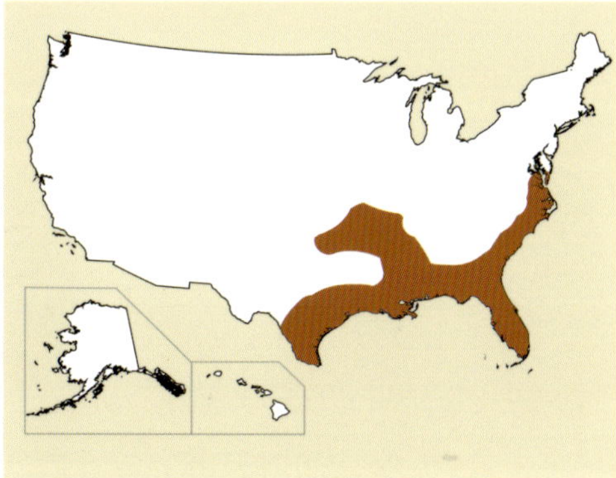

Figure 15. Distribution of Gulf Coast tick (*A. maculatum*) in the United States.

Dermacentor spp.

There are several species of *Dermacentor* ticks that have an impact on dogs and cats [Fig. 16, Table 4].

Table 4. *Dermacentor* ticks and their common names.

Species	Name
D. variabilis	American dog tick
D. andersoni	Rocky Mountain wood tick
D. reticulatus	Ornate dog tick Meadow tick

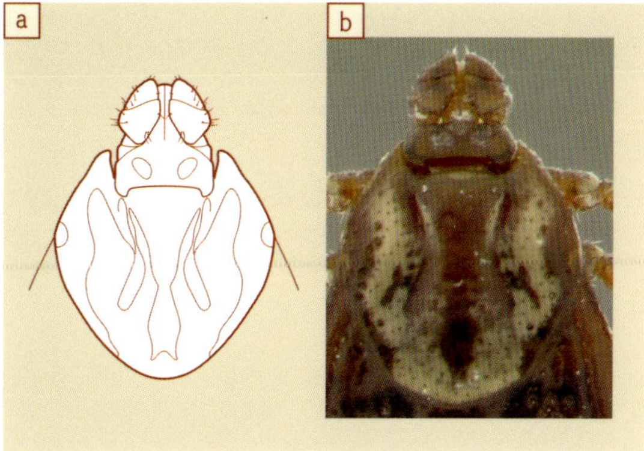

Figure 16. (a) Diagram and (b) photo of the head and scutum of *Dermacentor* spp. Image courtesy of Lyle J. Buss, Entomology and Nematology Department, University of Florida, US.

Both *D. variabilis* [American dog tick, Fig. 17] and *D. andersoni* [Rocky Mountain wood tick, Fig. 18] are very common in the United States. Their distribution is illustrated in Figures 19 and 20.

D. variabilis **is one of the most commonly noted ticks in the United States.**

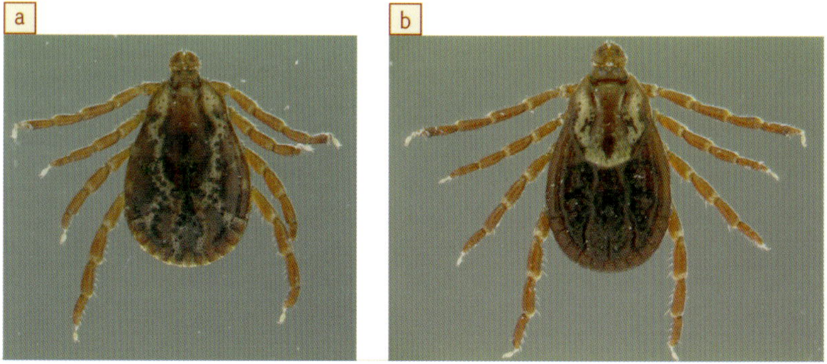

Figure 17. *D. variabilis*. (a) Male. (b) Female. Image courtesy of Lyle J. Buss, Entomology and Nematology Department, University of Florida, US.

a

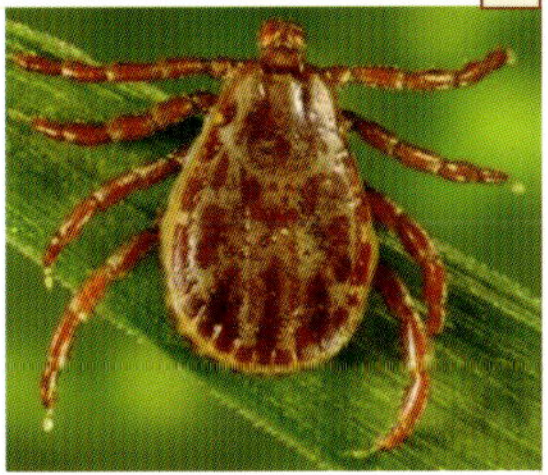

b

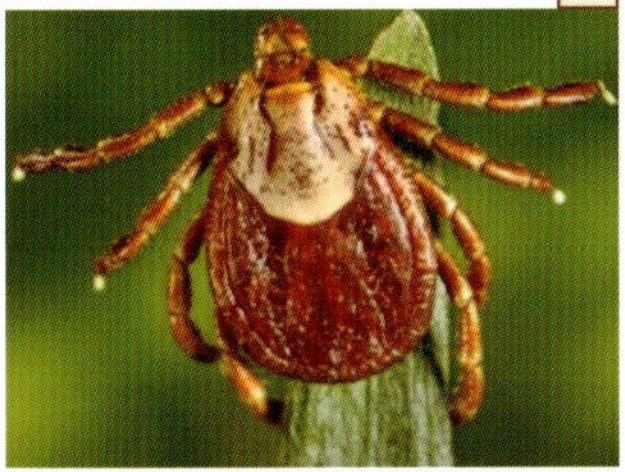

Figure 18.
D. andersoni.
(a) Male.
(b) Female.
Images courtesy of James Gathany, CDC.

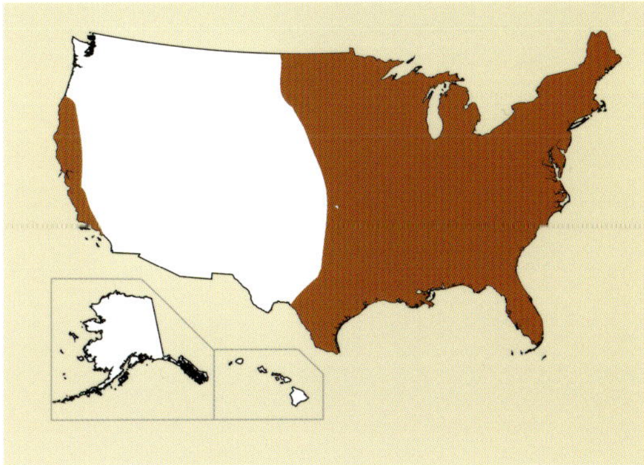

Figure 19. Distribution of American dog tick (*D. variabilis*) in the United States.

D. reticulatus is very widespread in Europe [Fig. 21].

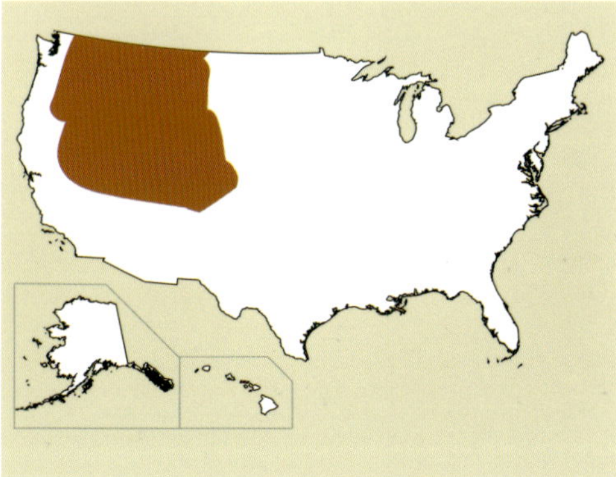

Figure 20. Distribution of Rocky Mountain wood tick (*D. andersoni*) in the United States.

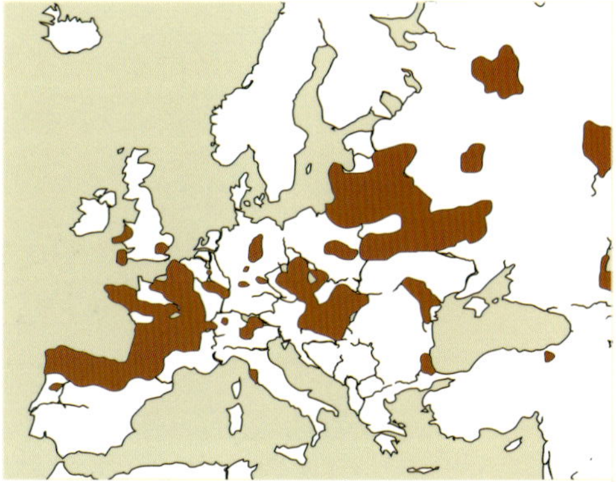

Figure 21. Distribution of ornate dog tick (*D. reticulatus*) in Europe and Near East.

As all the hard ticks species reviewed in this work, *Dermacentor* spp. is a 3-host tick. *D. variabilis* life stages are detailed in Table 5. It most commonly targets smaller mammals as a larva and nymph, and larger mammals – including dogs, cattle, horses, and even humans – as an adult.

Table 5. Life stages of *D. variabilis*.

Stage	Dimensions	Aspect	Comments
Larvae	0.6 mm long	Light brown/yellow	Feed for 2-14 days; molt over 7 days or more; can survive 11 months without feeding.
Nymph	0.9 mm long	Yellow to brown	Feed for 3-10 days; molt over 3 weeks to months; can survive 6 months without feeding.
Adult male (see Fig. 17a)	3.6 mm long	Red-brown, gray-silver markings on scutum	Can survive up to 2 years without feeding.
Adult female (see Fig. 17b)	5 mm long	Red-brown, gray-silver markings on scutum	Feed for 4-14 days; can survive up to 2 years without feeding.
Engorged female	15 mm long, 10 mm wide	Gray, silver/gray on scutum helps with identification	Can lay 4,000-7,000 eggs before dying.

Ixodes spp.

Ixodes ticks [Fig. 22] are well known due to association with the transmission of Lyme disease (*Borrelia burgdorferi*, see Table 10). Common names based on species are listed in Table 6.

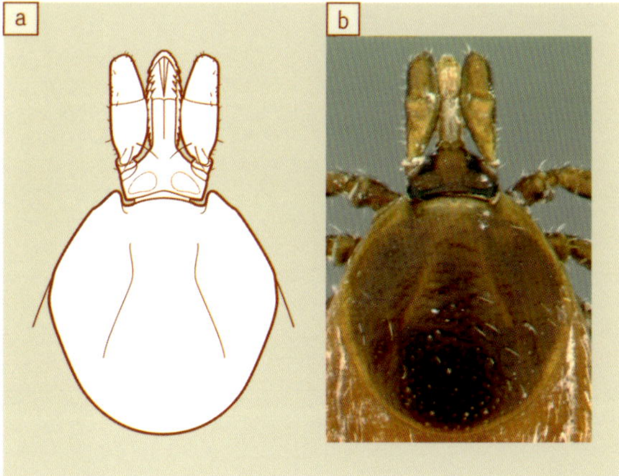

Figure 22. (a) Diagram and (b) photo of the head and scutum of *Ixodes* spp. Image courtesy of Lyle J. Buss, Entomology and Nematology Department, University of Florida, US.

Table 6. *Ixodes* ticks and their common names.

Species	Name
I. scapularis	Deer tick Blacklegged tick
I. pacificus	Western blacklegged tick
I. ricinus	European wood tick Castor bean tick Sheep tick
I. holocyclus	Australian paralysis tick

The pathogen that causes Lyme disease is transmitted by *Ixodes* ticks and maintained by wild small mammal reservoirs (especially rodents).

Whereas *I. scapularis* [Fig. 23] is more present in the East Coast, *I. pacificus* [Fig. 24] is more frequently seen in the West Coast. Their distribution is illustrated in Figures 25 and 26.

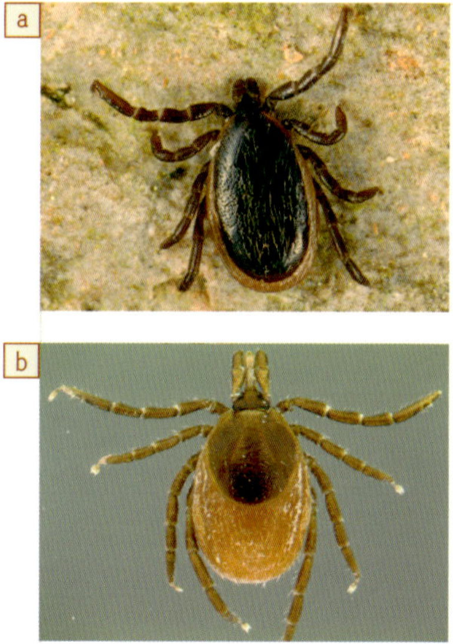

Figure 23. *I. scapularis.* (a) Male. (b) Female. Image courtesy of Lyle J. Buss, Entomology and Nematology Department, University of Florida, US.

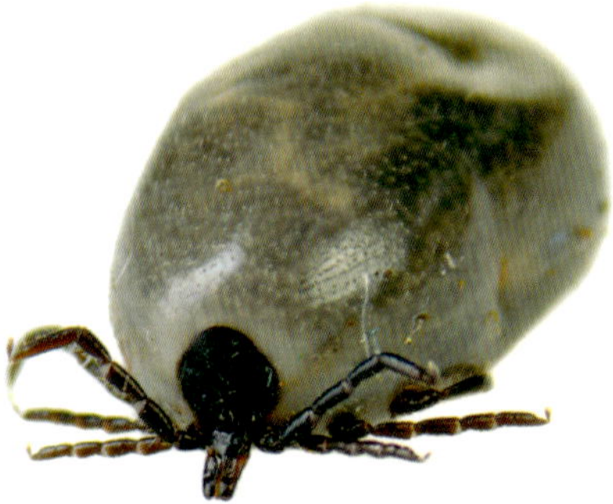

Figure 24. Western black-legged tick (*I. pacificus*) a few days after engorging blood from a dog. Image by Jeffrey B. Banke/shutterstock.com.

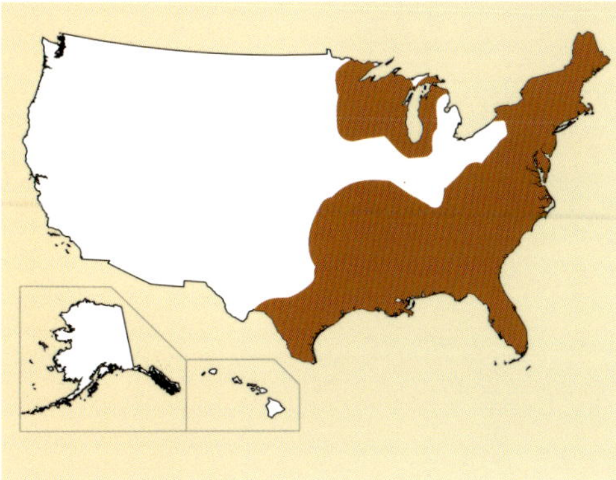

Figure 25. Distribution of deer tick (*I. scapularis*) in the United States.

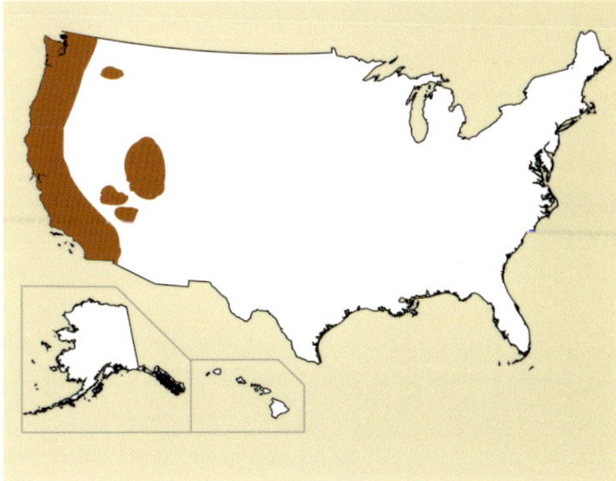

Figure 26. Distribution of western blacklegged tick (*I. pacificus*) in the United States.

In Europe, *I. ricinus* is the most common and widely spread hard tick in Europe [Figs. 27 and 28].

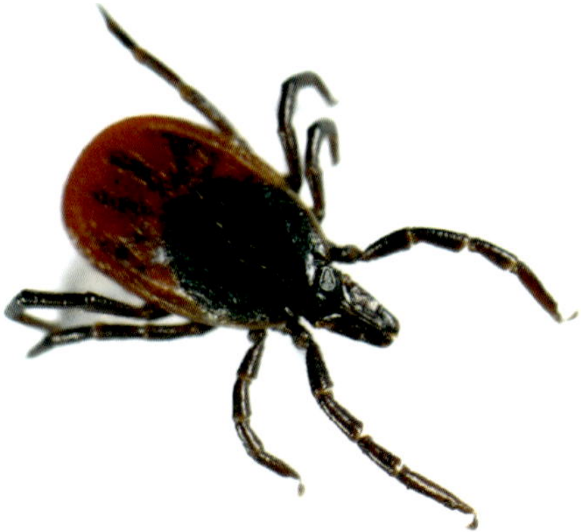

Figure 27. *I. ricinus* tick. Image by D. Kucharski K. Kucharska/shutterstock.com.

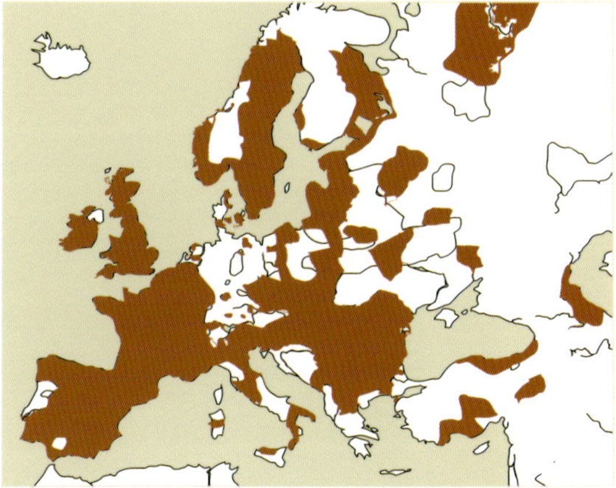

Figure 28. Distribution of castor bean tick (*I. ricinus*) in Europe.

I. scapularis larvae and nymphs feed on small mammals and birds. Adults feed on larger mammals and, occasionally, on humans [Table 7].

Table 7. Life stages of *I. scapularis.*			
Stage	**Dimensions**	**Aspect**	**Comments**
Larvae	1 mm long or less	White to light brown	Feed for 3-5 days.
Nymph	2 mm long or less	Light brown	Feed for 3-4 days.
Adult male (see Fig. 23a)	3 mm long	Dark brown to black; no festoons	Rarely feed.
Adult female (see Fig. 23b)	3-5 mm long	Orange-reddish brown with dark brown/black scutum	Feed for 5-7 days.
Engorged female	Up to 1 cm long	Grey with dark brown/black, round scutum visible	Lay 1,000-3,000 eggs.

In Australia, one of the most medically significant species is *I. holocyclus*. These ticks are most frequently encountered in the Australian East coast [Figs. 29 and 30]. As this area also contains the majority of Australia's population, pet and human infestations are relatively common.

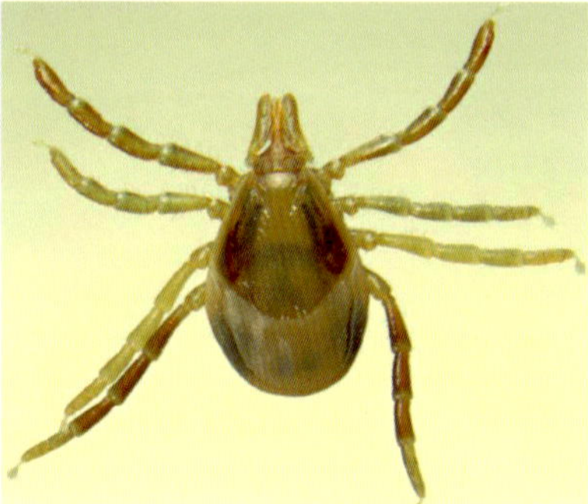

Figure 29. *I. holocyclus*. Note the darker front and rear legs, representative of this species.

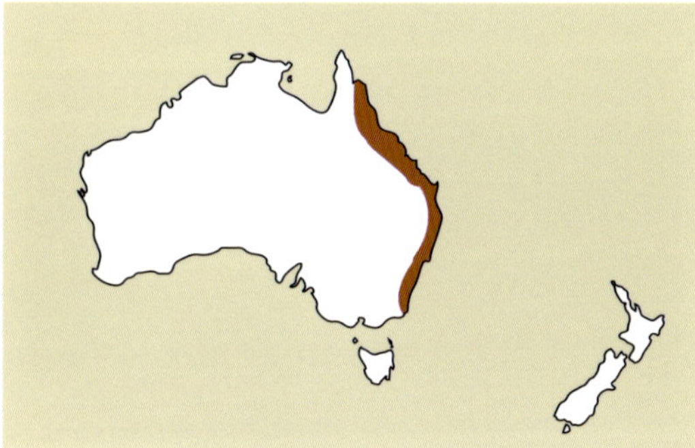

Figure 30. Australian paralysis tick distribution.

Haemaphysalis longicornis

H. longicornis' primary host is cattle, but has been found on other large and small mammals, including dogs, and also on birds [Fig. 31]. Common names vary based on geographical areas [Table 8].

Table 8. Common names for *H. longicornis*.

Area	Common name
Australia	Scrub tick, bush tick
New Zealand	Cattle tick

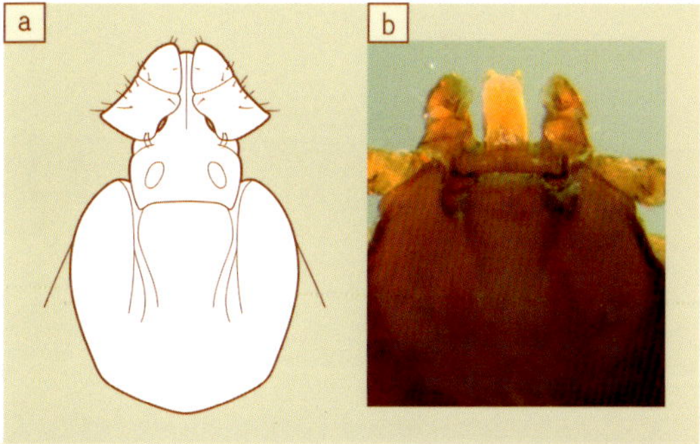

Figure 31. (a) Diagram and (b) photo of the head and scutum of *H. longicornis*. Note the short mouth parts. Image courtesy of Dr. Julia Kasper, New Zealand Biosecure Entomology Lab.

Table 9. Life stages of *H. longicornis*

Stage	Dimensions	Aspect	Comments
Larvae	0.6 mm long	Yellow to light brown	Feed for 3-9 days.
Nymph	Up to 2 mm long	Brown	Feed for 3-8 days.
Adult male	3 mm long	Reddish brown, festoons	
Adult female [Fig. 32]	3 mm long	Reddish brown, brown scutum, festoons	Feed for 7-14 days.
Engorged female	Up to 10 mm long	Gray with yellow striations	May lay 2000 eggs.

H. longicornis is found along the Eastern and Western coasts of Australia, Northern New Zealand, as well as parts of Japan and Eastern China [Fig. 32].

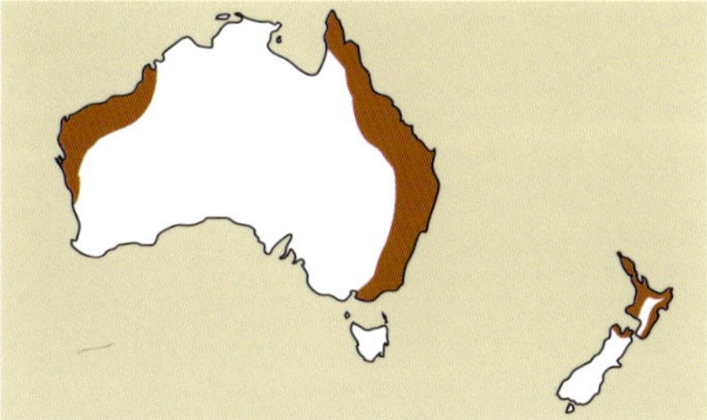

Figure 32. New Zealand cattle tick distribution.

Table 10. Tick-borne diseases.

Pathogen	Disease	Tick vector	Geographic distribution	Clinical findings
Anaplasma phagocytophilum	Anaplasmosis	*Ixodes* spp., *Rhipicephalus, Haemaphysalis*	Worldwide	Fever, lethargy, anorexia, musculoskeletal pain
Borrelia burgdorferi	Lyme	*Ixodes* spp., *Haemaphysalis* (possible)	North America, Europe, Asia	Fever, anorexia, musculoskeletal pain (often shifting legs), polyarthritis, lymph node enlargement, acute renal failure
Babesia canis canis	Babesiosis	*Dermacentor reticulatus*	Europe	Fever, hemolytic anemia
Babesia canis vogeli	Babesiosis	*Rhipicephalus sanguineus*	Worldwide	Fever, thrombocytopenia, anemia

Ehrlichia canis	Canine monocytotropic ehrlichiosis	*Rhipicephalus sanguineus*	Worldwide (except Australia)	Fever, anorexia, thrombocytopenia, anemia, central nervous system (CNS) signs, lymph node and splenic enlargement, uveitis, polyarthritis
Ehrlichia chaffeensis	Human monocytotropic ehrlichiosis	*Amblyomma americanum, Dermacentor variabilis*	Southern United States	Uveitis, vomiting, epistaxis, lymph node enlargement, thrombocytopenia
Rickettsia rickettsii	Rocky Mountain spotted fever (RMSF)	*Dermacentor, Amblyomma, Rhipicephalus*	North and South America	Fever, ocular signs, edema, lymph node enlargement, hemorrhage, musculoskeletal pain, CNS signs, dyspnea
Rickettsia conorii	Boutonneuse/ Mediterranean spotted fever	*Rhipicephalus sanguineus, Dermacentor reticulatus*	Mediterranean, Middle East, Africa	Similar to RMSF

Pathogen	Disease	Tick vector	Geographic distribution	Clinical findings
Francisella tularensis	Tularemia	*Dermacentor andersoni, Dermacentor variabilis, Amblyomma americanum*	North America (biting flies are more common vectors in Europe)	Cats more susceptible than dogs Fever, marked depression, enlarged lymph nodes, oral ulcers, icterus
Hepatozoon canis	Hepatozoonosis	*Rhipicephalus sanguineus*	Tropical, subtropical and temperate climates worldwide	Fever, anemia, lethargy, weight loss
Hepatozoon americanum	Hepatozoonosis	*Amblyomma maculatum*	Southern United States	Gait abnormalities, anemia, fever, lethargy, hyperesthesia
Tick salivary neurotoxins	Tick paralysis	*Dermacentor variabilis, D. andersoni, Amblyomma americanum, A. maculatum, Ixodes* spp.	Worldwide	Rapid, ascending paresis to paralysis

Otobius megnini

The spinose ear tick [*Otobius megnini*, Figs. 33 and 34] is one of very few soft ticks of clinical significance in dogs and cats. It is typically noted in livestock, but has been known to parasitize dogs and, rarely, cats.

The tick can be found throughout the Southern and Western United States. The occurrence in other areas of the country is usually due to the transportation of livestock. This tick has also been reported in other countries throughout the world.

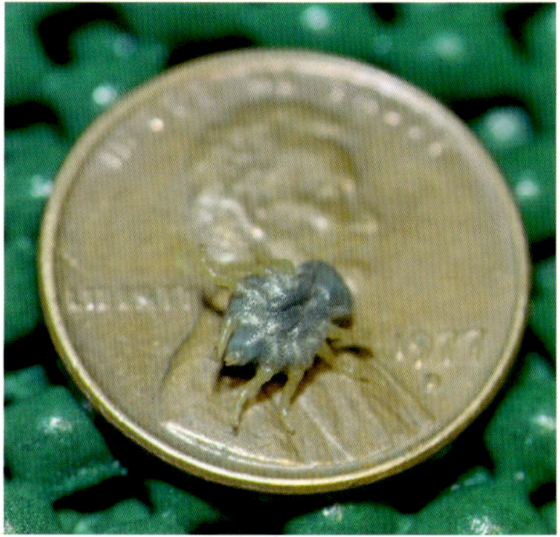

Figure 33. *O. megnini*. Image courtesy of Richard Meadow, DVM, DABVP, University of Missouri, US.

The larval and nymphal stages are parasitic but the adults do not feed on the host. After hatching, the immature stages travel to ear canals to feed and molt. Larvae molt to a nymphal stage which then molt to a second nymphal stage. After feeding, the second stage leaves the ear and molts to the adult stage. Mating occurs outside the ear canal; females will lay several batches of eggs before dying off [Table 11].

O. megnini is a one-host tick, meaning that all stages take place on the same host.

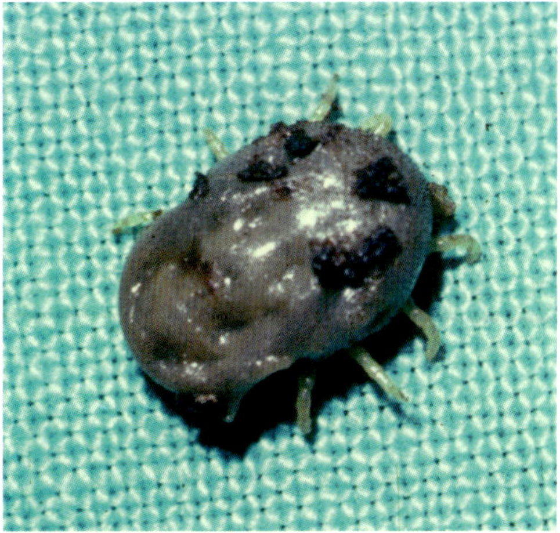

Figure 34. *O. megnini* removed from canine ear canal. Image courtesy of Stephen White, DVM, DACVD, UC Davis, US.

Table 11. Life stages of *O. megnini.*

Stage	Dimensions	Aspect	Comments
Larvae	0.5 mm long	Yellow-pink, spherical body, 3 pairs of legs	Can survive 2-4 months without feeding.
Nymph (first stage)	Up to 4 mm long	Blue-gray wide body with sharp spines, yellow legs	Feed for about 1 month.
Nymph (second stage)	Up to 8 mm long	Blue-gray wide body with sharp spines, yellow legs	Feed for 1-7 months.
Adults	Up to 10 mm long	Constricted in the middle (violin- shaped) with no spines	Females may lay eggs for up to 6 months.

While *O. megnini* infestation may be asymptomatic, it can lead to ear canal irritation and otitis. The otitis may extend to the middle ear in severe cases.

Tick removal

Ticks should never be removed with fingers as this could lead to transmission of tick-borne diseases.

Ticks should be extracted using pointed tweezers, hemostats [Fig. 35], or a tool designed specifically for tick removal. These instruments will allow the head of the tick to be grasped at the level of the host's skin.

Once grasped, the tick should be pulled in an upward, firm, and steady motion. Any twisting motion could result in incomplete removal or tearing of the tick's head.

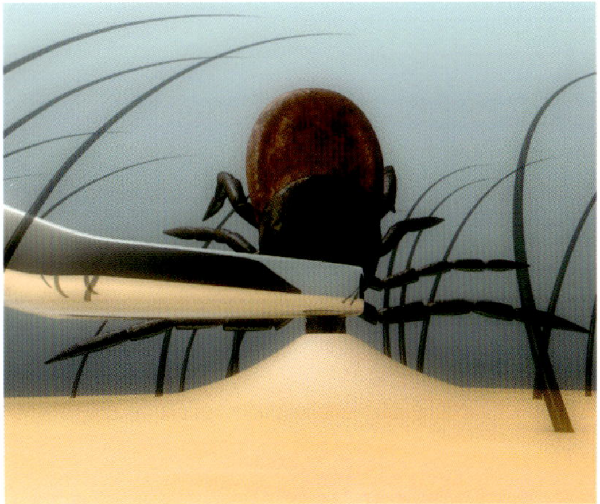

Figure 35. Tick removal using hemostats. Image by Sebastian Kaulitzki/shutterstock.

7 Prevention

Because the majority of the tick's life cycle is spent off-host, environmental control is as important as treating the host. This includes treating yards, perimeters of houses as well as inside. Keeping landscaping clear of debris and preventing wildlife from entering the environment can also be helpful.

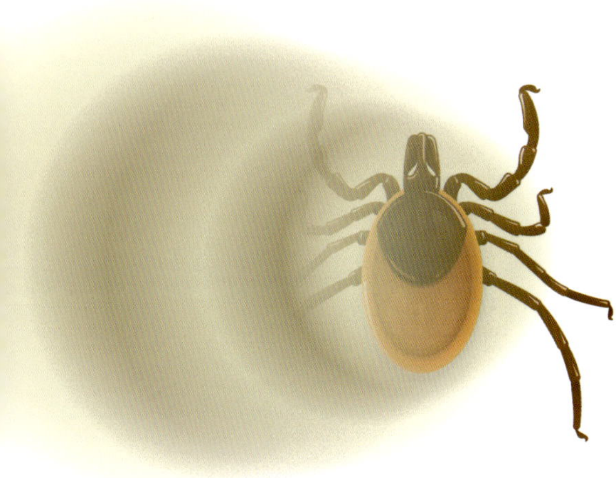

Insecticides, repellents and growth regulators to treat the environment and hosts are recommended. The process can take months to completely clear an infestation.

8 References

BLAGBURN BL, DRYDEN MW. Biology, Treatment, and Control of Flea and Tick Infestations. *Vet Clin Small Anim*. 2009, 39:1173-1200.

DANTAS-TORRES F. The brown dog tick, *Rhipicephalus sanguineus* (Latreille, 1806) (Acari: Ixodidae). From taxonomy to control. *Veterinary Parasitology*. 2008, 152:173-185.

GODDARD J, VARELA-STOKES A. Role of the lone star tick, *Amblyomma americanum* (L.), in human and animal diseases. *Veterinary Parasitology*. 2009, 160:1-12.

GREENE, CE. Infectious Diseases of the Dog and Cat, 4th ed Elsevier. 2012.

MILLER WH, GRIFFIN CE, CAMPBELL KL. Muller & Kirk's Small Animal Dermatology, 7th ed Elsevier. 2013, 294-295.

RICHTER D, MATUSCHKA FR, SPIELMAN A *et al*. How ticks get under your skin: insertion mechanics of the feeding apparatus of *Ixodes ricinus* ticks. *Proc R Soc B*. 2013, 280.

STRICKLAND RK, GERRISH RR, HOURRIGAN JL et al. Ticks of Veterinary Importance. *APHIS/USDA Agriculture Handbook*. 1976, 485:1-122.

WALKER K. Australian paralysis tick (*Ixodes holocyclus*). 2006, available online: PaDIL - http://www.padil.gov.au.

Internet resources

http://www.cdc.gov/ticks/

http://csu-cvmbs.colostate.edu/

http://entnemdept.ufl.edu/

http://ecdc.europa.eu/en/healthtopics/vectors/Pages/vectors.aspx

http://www.smsl.co.nz/site/southernmonitoring/files/NZB/Ha%20longicornis%20Profile.pdf

http://www.tandfonline.com/doi/abs/10.1080/00480169.2015.1035769#.VZ23H_lViko

http://thewww.lowchensaustralia.com/pests/paralysis-tick/ixodes-holocyclus-description.htm

http://www.padil.gov.au/pests-and-diseases/pest/main/136496